Brain

Training

How To Unlock Your Hidden Potential

(The Ultimate Guide to Discovering the Power of Your Brain and Improving Your Memory)

Chris Deroche

Published By **Jackson Denver**

Chris Deroche

Brain Training: How To Unlock Your Hidden Potential (The Ultimate Guide to Discovering the Power of Your Brain and Improving Your Memory)

ISBN 978-1-998927-63-0

Legal & Disclaimer

The information contained in this book is not designed to replace or take the place of any form of medicine or professional medical advice. The information in this book has been provided for educational & entertainment purposes only.

The information contained in this book has been compiled from sources deemed reliable, and it is accurate to the best of the Author's knowledge; however, the Author cannot guarantee its accuracy and validity and cannot be held liable for any errors or omissions. Changes are periodically made to this book. You must consult your doctor or get professional medical advice before using any of the suggested remedies, techniques, or information in this book.

Table Of Contents

Chapter 1: Train Your Brain Or Else.......... 1

Chapter 2: How To Train Your Brain......... 9

Chapter 3: It Is Also Fun!........................ 17

Chapter 4: Making Your Brain Sharp 27

Chapter 5: Is There Such Thing As Brain
Fitness?.. 36

Chapter 6: The Power Of Brain Training. 48

Chapter 7: What Is Brain Training And Why
It Matters? 55

Chapter 8: How Workout Trains The
Thoughts? 72

Chapter 9: Good Habits For The Brain.... 95

Chapter 10: Feed Your Brain - Keep Your
Mind 131

Chapter 11: Can You Reverse Memory
Loss? 152

Chapter 1: Train Your Brain Or Else

We all recognize that the mind is the center of the aggravating device of vertebrate and invertebrate creatures on this worldwide. Today, we're going to attention on the Human Brain. Even despite the fact that the mind is most effective a 3 pound spongy organ inside our skull, it's miles the middle of intelligence, manages our senses, and controls our body actions and behavior. The thoughts performs a vital characteristic in our device; consequently, it ought to be looked after. A part of statistics how to attend to our thoughts, method we also want to train our mind at times. Yes, even our thoughts dreams training (no longer just our muscle groups).

• Let's Define Brain Training

Brain Training is described as a simple workout to decorate and beautify the capacity to adapt, learn abruptly, and more without troubles. The brain has what we call neurons, which device the records from a compound network. While we are within the process of getting to know, the ones neurons art work as a difficult and speedy to finish gaining knowledge of and carry out the responsibilities. As we adapt and analyze, the ones businesses of neurons paintings as one to complete the questioning duties. There are such a number of strategies and assessments on how we are able to teach our mind.

These mind education tests are designed for each shape of man or woman. Some thoughts training assessments may be used by all varieties of humans and a few are designed for precise personalities. There are severa dreams who acquired't possibly have the same response to the identical mind-training assessments which includes healthy kids, teenagers, adults, older adults, adults with mid mind impairment, adults with demanding mind harm, and older adults with dementia or top notch types of brain ailments.

Did that mind education businesses have loved large fulfillment within the past years? Yes they have got, and there are loads of lots of customers for the ones mind training programs round the world.

Most researchers actually pick out out a category or from those businesses to reputation on. When they're accomplished with the administration of the brain education, they need to have a look at the effects one after the alternative because of the fact they're targeted on brilliant businesses from our population.

People say that thoughts schooling or cognitive training can assist self improvement. The mechanism of thoughts education is that new facts turns into information at the equal time as it's far absorbed with the resource of the person's cognitive talents which includes reminiscence and seen processing or now and again auditory processing. The electricity in mind training is determined by way of its functionality to apprehend the purpose and fortify the person's talents.

Cognitive competencies, including revel in processing, memory, hobby, and reasoning additionally can be advanced with the right training. With this education for our mind, there can be much more likely an immediate response from the mind's function, memory strengthens, processing of records will become quicker, or quicker absorption of latest understanding and much less complicated complete response throughout a big preference of such mastering worrying conditions. Brain training furthermore strengthens and complements the cognitive competencies of an person, which actually permits the device of analyzing to be extra a success and run effortlessly. The secret to this is being capable of determine or find out the proper thoughts device efficiently.

For the longest time, psychologists had been looking to make the intelligence of humans expand faster. There are also research approximately the walking reminiscence capability of an individual being particularly related to complicated analyzing and hobby manipulate, even which encompass trouble fixing. But we ought to understand that when the memory capacity internal your thoughts increases, it does not imply that the volume of your intelligence moreover will increase. To date, there are numerous research that display the benefits of thoughts schooling, but handiest a couple of these tests have examined the variation of these to our regular lives.

Brain training consequences are constrained to the proper tasks being taught and cannot be generalized to unique obligations or cognitive features. There also are net-primarily based definitely actually thoughts education alternatives which do not look like significantly diverse in final results from traditional pencil and paper-primarily based schooling, but then, the benefits of those are exertions financial savings and efficiency will increase.

Brain education will not make you a genius or smarter than others, however it's going to make you perform higher and enhance whatever exercise you execute. Just go through in thoughts, you'll constantly get better at some aspect you do repetitively. You can't hold close a assignment by manner of in search of to do it simply as speedy as. A mission we perform a pair times will not offer us an immediate and unique quit end result. The brain can reduce or thicken, plus neural links can be copied and evolved or from time to time weaken based on tremendous environmental conditions. There is continually what we name exercising and this is one issue we need to never neglect about so as for our thoughts to continuously mature and boom.

More and further evi-dence indicates and proves that mind train-ing can paintings. The ques-tion is, how-ever, how can we maximize the ones education durations, and adapt them to our every day life?

• Use Your Brain!

Studies have established that the mind is continuously changing and evolving. This technique that the grey remember quantity internal our skull keeps to broaden so long as we're alive. Once we workout and use our mind, our Intelligence Quotient or IQ will develop and enhance on the identical time. A researcher stated that the more lively we are, the greater neurons in our brains are forming specially inside the reminiscence manage place. Also, residing an energetic way of life continues the tissues in our mind lively as well. Tell me, who couldn't need to have a healthy and beneficial mind? And we realize for a reality that if some element isn't getting used or mobilized, it gets rusty and breaks on its very very own. So, manifestly we do not need our thoughts to get rusty and in fact save you running on its private due to the fact we don't use it, right? We absolutely want to apply and workout our mind in order for us to decorate what we've got got already received as we age and make sure that the records we've can be useful in our each day lives. That is why it's miles crucial that we educate our mind sometimes.

Chapter 2: How To Train Your Brain

What is Brain Exercise? Brain exercise will permit you to growth and enhance your memory, interest, and alertness.

We are too busy going to art work, university, and doing our each day sports, and we forget about approximately to enhance our brains, permit it loosen up and permit it beautify in a natural manner. Our brains are going for walks all the time, it's miles up to us to ensure we're able to have a pointy memory and preserve it walking nicely.

It's a fantastic concept to get exercise in your thoughts every so often, you've got no longer some thing to lose. Most in all likelihood, you don't need to spend a unmarried penny for it. There are a whole lot of thoughts sporting events that you may do from the consolation your own home, and you can even invite a pal to join you, to make it extra fun!

So, proper right right here are the smooth sporting events that we are capable of do on every occasion and everywhere: study greater to find out!

1. Writing

Believe it or not, writing is an powerful easy manner to exercise our mind. By surely writing, we're able to stimulate the way of wondering. Writing takes the left part of our mind so we're in a function to test our spelling, grammar, and any descriptive facts.

2. Play video video video games

Yes, that could be a fun however a simple way to workout your thoughts. You can play video video games like simulations, puzzles, or maybe an movement sport. This is an possibility to workout your choice-making competencies, as it lets in us to remember the extremely good viable approach to a problem. Aside from this, we're capable of exercising our eye movement and hand eye coordination as we play video video video games.

3. Play an tool

You in all likelihood understand the way to play guitar, piano, or drums. Why no longer use your abilities to exercising your mind? It can provide you with a entire mind workout from listening to, sight, and touch.

four. Play sports sports

Playing sports can be some thing from soccer, volleyball, or even playing a smooth basketball activity to your outdoor. It indicates that those those who are actively gambling sports activities have larger brains and feature super hobby capabilities. Also, it's going to assist us to be extra energetic and will assist you sleep higher.

five. Have enough sleep

Sleeping is part of our each day everyday, but a few human beings can also forget that dozing is vital for a human. Yes, mainly a person who works more than complete time hours and a person who works at night. Sleeping is important for productivity, reading, and reminiscence function of our brains.

6. Learn New Skills

Any new abilties which you have now not observed however may be a excellent start, you could both enrol in a class or observe on your non-public. Learning new talents is a extremely good workout for our thoughts's creativity feature. Our mind works in a ordinary, which includes a similarly set of skills gets your mind sharper.

So, those are only a few easy physical video video games that you could do to your own or along with your pal. There are virtually lots of wearing activities, however it usually is based upon if we have time and if we are excessive approximately workout our brains for better and sharper productiveness.

•Examples

Now that we have were given study a few easy sporting activities that we will do on our very very own, we already have thoughts approximately the potential and the way are we able to attain it. So those are just a few examples of easy physical games: Read on to discover more!

Grab a newspaper. A newspaper is a fantastic manner to workout your thoughts because it consists of multiple topics from politics, to buying, and celebrities. Read as lots as you may and get your thoughts jogging out, mainly within the morning because of the reality this could get it revved as a great deal as paintings nicely at a few level within the day.

Let's play chess! Chess is a totally complex recreation for novices, but take word: this is the most effective pastime in case you need an workout for your thoughts. Chess can stimulate some of our thoughts capabilities from memory to choice-making abilties. There's lots to have a look at in the starting, however there may be plenty to benefit on the identical time as playing chess.

Take a dictionary. A dictionary consists a whole lot of words, terms which is probably familiar to us and phrases that are not. It isn't a horrible idea to take some time coming across new terms, it can assist beautify our reminiscence and preserve new statistics that can be useful for our vocabulary. Our vocabulary is constrained to what we are pronouncing and what we know, but analyzing new phrases can boom our facts and improve our self confidence.

Enrol your self in a class! Learning need to not save you at the same time as we graduate from university, it want to be a non-forestall way in the route of our lives. So, enrolling your self in a category which you're involved in, whether or not it's far a tune elegance or a yoga class, it's miles a tremendous exercise for our thoughts. Aside from getting to know, we can also educate our brains by socializing. Being part of a hard and fast is amusing, you enjoy learning and socializing with people who percentage the same hobby.

Learn a modern day language! If you are a close-by English speaker, then studies the Chinese language. You can enrol in a language elegance or you can even locate on line instructions if you locate your time table is just too tight. You also can really purchase a ebook of your desired language and observe at your personal tempo, it's far a tough exercise however don't forget all that you may benefit from learning a extremely-modern-day language.

Play your tool! Playing your device can be fun and on the identical time it is an workout for our thoughts. Just hold close your guitar, piano, or any available tool in your private home, then play a music that you recognise. Don't apprehend the way to play your tool? Not a hassle, there are hundreds of films on line that you can discover very useful, specifically for novices, they show a grade by grade system for playing your tool.

Brain sports activities ought to now not be high-priced, you can be modern, and there are probably masses of materials internal of your own home. Also, these sporting sports activities are meant to assist us enhance our brains and be the excellent individual that we can be. You also can discover this beneficial in case you hit your forty's or 50's in which maximum humans will be inclined to forget approximately some subjects approximately their each day everyday. Again, it's far just all approximately being energetic and taking properly care of our brains for our personal health gain.

Chapter 3: It Is Also Fun!

Just including you do a work out to physically get your frame in form, your brain furthermore desires a schooling ordinary to be at its pinnacle of alertness. The maxim "use it or lose it" holds real in this situation. The more you operate your thoughts for effective thinking, the greater you becomes an alert, centered, and inexperienced philosopher. There are masses of things that can be finished so one can sharpen your cognitive energy. Some of them might be too apparent to state, at the equal time as others may be too bizarre to attempt. But irrespective of how the habitual can also additionally seem to you, all of it boils all the way all the way down to a unmarried goal, and that is, of direction, to enhance your intellectual functionality.

This chapter will talk a few a laugh strategies or techniques that you may without difficulty do to exercise your thoughts and to keep your self mentally healthful. Scientifically talking our thoughts is characterised with the beneficial aid of number one additives of cognitive functions which consist of: memory, interest, perception, motor, language, visible-spatial processing, and government talents. All the ones skills are of equal significance in keeping amazing cognition. Below are some discussions that would manual you in placing your mental health in fine fettle.

Memory at paintings

Yes, you heard it proper. Working your reminiscence out continues to be the exceptional element you can do as a manner to maintain cognitive fog away. Scientists display that our mind is basically sharpened through the movements of the chemical compound that triggers mind cell repair called acetylcholine. So maintaining the amount of this chemical on your mind let you maintain that laser-like reminiscence.

Food for notion

Eating healthful is the primary huge key that defines an powerful workout ordinary in your mind. Remember that you have to boost your acetylcholine degree for you to facilitate appropriate memory skills. This may be completed through eating elements wealthy in Omega-three fatty acids, which can be derived from fish and nuts. Research furthermore shows that dark chocolate, rich in flavanols – an antioxidant that sustains active neuron characteristic, can beneficial aid us to hold right memory.

Reading is learning

Our reminiscence may be categorically labeled into kinds: quick-time period and long time. Short term memory or energetic reminiscence is the functionality of your mind to maintain specific quantities of data for a short time period. Long time period memory, rather, is the functionality to hold statistics for longer intervals. Reading is thought to be the handiest manner of improving our reminiscence. Depending on the nature of textual content we are studying, our thoughts can hold information for a quick time or an extended time. Repetition is also a way that could help us keep statistics in our reminiscence. This is the reason why we understand signage very well due to the reality we come across them on a every day basis.

Brain schooling application

A business enterprise of neuroscientists from Stanford University in collaboration with the University of California advanced a training course this is called "Lumosity". This is a mind hobby that can be accessed thru the internet or may be downloaded for your mobile devices, which includes varying tiers of a series of video games that energize memory functions. This may be an powerful tool to preserve your brain challenged.

Keep your hobby keen

Attention and notion are two important additives of an important whole. These are cognitive abilties that paintings hand in hand in growing better mental competencies. The method includes eager recognition of sensory stimuli and the capability to maintain your attention on a selected aspect, perception, or movement amidst numerous distractions.

Perceive and be attentive

Attention is full-size in our each day residing. Paying hobby to a particular trouble do not forget permits your thoughts to understand each the overall and specific information that are had to apprehend the totality of that mission. Perception is vital as nicely because it adds the important coordination of your body elements, specially your senses, to paintings coherently in comprehending a specific outdoor stimulus.

Ability to multi-mission

You can do smooth bodily games that allows you to maintain your interest and perception green, which consist of doing all of your math whilst typing, or memorizing tune lyrics on the same time as taking a jog. These shifts in your mental panorama can certainly assist you neurons in associating particular neural connections at the identical time.

Gauge your language

Another critical feature of your cognitive capability is your language capacity. This allows you to associate terms to which means that, sounds, and phonetics to verbal outputs. Level up your language abilties with a few clean exercise drills.

Things you observe is understanding you benefit

One very commonplace manner to enhance your language skills is by using the usage of using analyzing loads. It is in analyzing that we come across terms that we are not acquainted with. List those phrases which can be new to you. Use the dictionary to look for their meanings and try to use them in your each day verbal exchange. That manner, you gain new information and also you increase your vocabulary.

Right detail in writing

Writing is also an method that can decorate your language capabilities. Once you write some thing, you think, and consider topics. There is always a vital region that hyperlinks up your writing and language capabilities. A character who can write efficaciously is a person who has entire data approximately what he writes. A well-versed man or woman is then a person who has enough language skills that he can reflect his mind comprehensively on a piece of paper.

Try new, speak new

Learning a brand new language is a completely apparent example to boom your language abilities. Once you attempt to research a contemporary language, you comprise yourself in a totally difficult environment. This way, you mission your mind to recognize and communicate a state-of-the-art language that may be an effective device in widening your sphere of socialization and interaction.

Not definitely the picture however the movement

Other cognitive functions which might be all similarly important to your intellectual health are motor abilties, seen-spatial processing, and the authorities competencies. These are liable for the general mobility and version to the prevailing outside stimuli.

In our every day lives, we're confronted with one-of-a-kind situations wherein we show our potential to cope with them through the use of taking the proper moves. This is a totally concrete instance that showcases the ability of your brain to machine trouble-fixing skills to provide you with the proper selections.

Get the strain to challenge yourself

Your motor skills may be stepped forward thru way of taking over greater stressful situations for yourself every so often. One clean example you could do is to update on your non-dominant hand at the identical time as doing all of your each day everyday activities. Try writing collectively together with your left hand if you're a right-surpassed person. Or try brushing your teeth collectively along with your proper hand if you are a left-exceeded character. This easy exercise can actually increase your brain's flexibility to replace from one mental mode to every exclusive, due to this developing new establishments in conjunction with your brain's neural composition.

Give your thoughts a chance to play

There are also a few brain traumatic conditions that you could try which might be to be had in the public area, much like the internet, that let you gather extra powerful visible-spatial capabilities, or even enhance your executive thoughts abilities. Video video games, due to the reality the studies indicates, aren't in fact that terrible. Studies claim that video video games are crucial equipment in growing strategies and problem solving skills. Or in case you are not an avid fan of that era, you may normally opt for the traditional mind teasers like Sudoku, puzzles, chess, and Rubik's dice which have same outcomes in maintaining your intellectual capability sharp. In something techniques you decided are applicable to you, remember that the reason you want to satisfy is to keep your thoughts challenged to stay centered and alert!

Chapter 4: Making Your Brain Sharp

Are you continue to sharp? --This is a query all people must solution because it displays the overall highbrow fitness of someone. However, some people generally tend to beat back the question, mainly at the identical time as symptoms of memory lapses start to kick in. The sharpness of the mind is important to survival. Without a doubt, a healthful memory is an critical parameter in defining our widespread fitness, our functionality to feature nicely, our cognitive ordinary typical performance, and even our mortality.

So yet again, how sharp are you? Our mind a long term similar to every organ of our body. The thoughts decreases in duration as we input the onset of adulthood. However, it additionally has the capability to develop. This happens if you deal with yourself properly and in case you include the basics of highbrow health for your regular existence.

Here are three smooth however effective strategies to show that your thoughts is, certainly, in top form:

1.Ability to keep in mind names and faces. This may also sound simple, but a number of humans, even at a extra younger age, have troubles recognizing faces and names. The conditions which envelop episodic memory lapses encompass forgetting of names, faces, or maybe smooth dates or celebrations. Sharp human beings are able to retrieve records pertaining to names and faces with out problems.

2.Ability to perform nice analytical functions mentally. Are you from time to time tempted to take out your small calculator at the same time as having to choose out the quantity you need to pay at the equal time as you skip Dutch? Are you capable of calculate positive smooth Mathematical problems right away? If you are despite the fact that capable of, then congratulations!

Your cognitive potential remains at a awesome degree.

three.Being happy and emotionally solid. Our thoughts is also liable for our emotions. Being emotionally strong is a sign of pinnacle mind function, which is also linked to regular intellectual abilties. If you're depressed or burdened, this should be addressed at once, as it could moreover abate your cognitive talents which might be responsible for your sharpness and reminiscence.

Needless to say, staying sharp can be appeared a primary tool for survival in addition to for durability. If you recognize someone with Alzheimer's ailment, you have got more reasons to take authentic care of your health. Older humans plagued with the said illness lose their cognitive abilties greater time, making it hard for them to function generally. If the thoughts keeps to decrease, even the only reminiscence of know-how how to stroll, take a bath, or even speech is going up in smoke. This is precisely why human beings with Dementia, in particular Alzheimer's, want a round-the-clock care.

Keeping your mind sharp isn't only a responsibility for older human beings. Beyond age, it's far predicated upon for your intellectual energy. Even extra younger human beings also can enjoy reminiscence lapses, but aren't truely privy to it. So no matter your age, you owe to yourself to make sure that your mind is healthy so that you can higher harness it, and advantage from its power.

If you're aiming to maintain your reminiscence sharper and your mind more healthy, you could do the subsequent hints:

Tip #01: Say good-bye to your sedentary manner of lifestyles. If you are certainly keen approximately turning over a modern day leaf, then you definately really in reality need to stay off the couch extra regularly.

Exercising and sweating it out at the least 20 minutes a day can enhance the oxygen diploma to your thoughts, which then moreover improves the capability of the mind to undergo in thoughts formerly encoded statistics. Furthermore, exercising additionally lets in in warding off illnesses that might purpose reminiscence impairment.

Tip#02: Do no longer isolate your self. Meet pals extra often. Better yet, be part of a membership or volunteer at an employer. Yes, that might be amusing. But greater importantly, spending time with pals and being socially active additionally helps in improving mind fitness. This, however, refers to individuals who are not engaged in social sports. People with a robust useful resource device and healthy social lives have little or no danger of growing cognitive decline. Depressed human beings are also greater susceptible to obtaining illnesses which consist of Dementia.

Tip #03. Ditch the beef. Have extra fish. Not best because it is the greater healthy choice, however because fish includes healthy oil called Omega-three which is good for thoughts development. You can also gain this wholesome oil in nuts and olives. So in case you are having problems considering what to consume for dinner, actually pick fish and you'll understand you are making an splendid choice.

Tip#04: Sleep well. Though this one is pretty obvious, you recognize that it's far tough to characteristic nicely in case you are sleep-deprived. Among the issues professional thru people who lack a normal amount of sleep is the decline in problem-fixing abilities, crucial thinking, and creative wondering. Sleep is crucial for the complete thoughts to work as it is also essential in maintaining the 'preserve in mind' feature at the circulate. Memory formation and consolidation additionally relies upon on first-rate sleep. It is, consequently, critical to avoid pulling an all-nighter often.

Tip #05: Get your mind operating. The mind desires regular responsibilities which encompass evaluation, critical questioning, and so forth to thrive. It is highly endorsed which you expand interests which may be connected with thoughts sports sports. For instance, doing pass-word puzzles, riddles, and studying are beneficial in retaining your mind lively. As with any tool, stagnant brainwork makes the memory rusty.

Tip#06. When careworn, try to meditate. Do no longer live on any annoying situation. Keep your strain diploma under manage, as it's far in truth one of the roadblocks to engaging in greater healthy memory. Stress can substantially harm a place in our mind known as the hippocampus- that is the principle unit of the thoughts that strategies encoded facts and maintains it in our reminiscence.

If you feel beneath an insurmountable amount of stress, it is encouraged which you strive precise tool for placing off it. One of the pretty encouraged equipment is through meditation. This does now not simplest cast off stress and boom reminiscence, it additionally permits enhance persistent conditions which are related to melancholy, excessive blood stress, and diabetes.

Tip #07. Got a telephone? Then use an app to absolutely zap the reminiscence decline away! We now live amidst a sea of programs inside the virtual international which may be mainly designed to maintain the mind functioning properly. Memory-boosting video games aren't best fun and precise, but moreover useful. If you aren't fantastic as to which app to download, you may seek advice from some seemed threads or on-line groups for opinions.

It is in no way too past due to start annoying in your mind!

Chapter 5: Is There Such Thing As Brain Fitness?

The phrase 'health' is frequently connected to the general fitness of the human frame. Regardless of age, gender, and age, people are required to be 'in shape' a high-quality manner to verify durability.

So the question is --are you physical healthful? You can effortlessly solution this with a easy YES or NO! The next question is – Is your mind healthy? Though it can startle you a piece to partner the thoughts with the phrase 'in form', it is wonderful that you may likely answer this with a powerful 'YES' as nicely.

But what precisely is 'Brain Fitness'?

If the human body thrives on bodily fitness, the human is sustained through what is known as 'Brain Fitness'. Though the analogy is simple, the precept in the back of the latter first got here into play about a few a long time in the past. Self-help books posted in 1989 -1990 included the time period 'Brain Fitness', which ultimately brought approximately a bout of Scientific studies to reveal its viability and feasibility.

To define the time period genuinely, Brain Fitness refers to having wholesome cognitive processing this is efficient, quick, and flexible. It is the by-product of in depth studies inside the fields of neuroscience and neuropsychology. To reap thoughts health, one has to preserve and train his cognitive abilties the use of clinical methods alongside aspect neurogenesis and neuroplasticity as the primary gadgets.

At present, many researchers within the in the meantime are on the quest for locating a measurable matrix that can be used to evaluate mind fitness at the physical degree. The process can also additionally encompass in depth take a look at of neurogenesis, and 'measuring' the wide type of synapse connections that broaden regularly or fast.

The dendrites linking the neurons also are one of the parameters of the matrices.

How is mind fitness completed?

1.Mental Simulation. You likely recognize through now that the brain includes hundreds and heaps of neurons which might be interconnected. Both the neurons and the connections may additionally moreover die through the years because of cellular death and incorrect care. Brain Fitness is evolved through way of way of encouraging the opposite to transpire. The regular cognitive dreams of everyday lifestyles push the producing of those neurons and strengthens their connectivity.

The impaired capacity of the thoughts cells to regenerate is the number one reason of cognitive decline, that could moreover cause extreme ailments such as dementia. Training for Brain Fitness was moreover performed thru manner of the Advanced Cognitive Training for Independent and Vital

Elderly (ACTIVE), the maximum essential business enterprise to conduct scientific studies on cognitive training for older humans. The outcomes of the clinical trials were posted inside the Journal of the American Medical Association again in 2002, revealing that older those who have been present process cognitive brain health schooling for five weeks had already demonstrated big development of their records processing, reasoning, and normal reminiscence.

2.By assignment severa mentally - challenging sports. Brain Fitness can also be finished via task numerous activities that may be both physical and mentally difficult. Playing chess, schooling yoga, or maybe laptop-based completely highbrow physical activities are amongst the usual examples. Doing puzzles and playing first-rate video video video games have moreover been used as systems for mind fitness. There are a developing variety of clubs and summer season camps for kids now which aren't handiest targeted on clean survival education, camping, and physical sports, but moreover encourage younger children to attempt chess, Sudoku, and plenty of others.

three.By formal training. Brain power additionally may be inspired to maintain it in shape thru formal schooling collectively with continuing schooling and taking new guides. By being mentally lively and constantly feeding your thoughts new records virtually prevents it from being rusty. Many retirees at the moment are turning into more and more interested by studying new talents to preserve their brains in top shape. There had been numerous studies studies that suggest development in highbrow fitness of people who choose to live mentally active regardless of having to go through other physical situations.

4.By retaining the bodily frame in shape as nicely. Choosing to live a extra healthy way of life is likewise pivotal to acquire intellectual fitness. People who do no longer fail to exercising, trust in particular nutrients, sleep well, and manipulate pressure stage effectively are a lot much less vulnerable to experiencing cognitive decline once they turn out to be older. This technique that a shielding protect in competition to dementia, Alzheimer's, and excessive despair is built through the years.

How does Brain Fitness help YOU?

Now which you understand how Brain Fitness is completed, it is time to investigate what its particular benefits are. You can also recognize via using now that every one cognitive abilities are superior with in form brains. But what exactly are we able to imply by using way of that. See the subsequent benefits to completely draw near how Brain Fitness can sincerely assist you:

•It keeps your reminiscence sharp. Gone are the instances while you drop incorrect names or are not able to apprehend the face of an acquaintance. Gone are the embarrassing moments of forgetting vital dates and activities.

•It lets in you get entry to your vocabulary quick. Lost for words? Maybe it is an example that you want to perform a few thoughts exercise exercises. Retrieval or bear in mind has a tendency to be extraordinarily tough if the thoughts gets rusty. This unique thing is critical for verbal exchange.

•It offers you sharper imaginative and prescient. The thoughts is also a essential hassle for your imaginative and prescient – no longer truely your eyes. With terrible brain health, recognizing a person in a crowded vicinity, the use of, and studying street symptoms all become a burden. Worse, terrible vision is also the diverse pinnacle reasons for injuries.

•It consequences in first-rate oral comprehension. Just like with vision, your taking note of's partner is likewise your mind. The capacity to recognize voices, recognize information clips, and being able to talk requires a first rate working thoughts.

•It makes you keep in mind you studied on your ft. This manner you may react and reply more rapid. You is probably capable of take in facts speedy that permits you to generate on the spot reactions. This is vital to your paintings, studies, or any challenge.

•It makes you a extra steady, notable driver. When using your whole mind energy at the equal time as using, you could store your self from the dangers of getting into an twist of future. How? This is because your mind receives to 'command' you proper away while matters do now not seem right.

•It makes you a pleasing individual. Your mood and everyday feelings additionally rely on how in shape or healthful your thoughts is. When you determine out the mind, it releases dopamine and unique chemical compounds that preserve you alert, satisfied, and excited.

•It boosts your self guarantee and vanity. Having a suit mind offers you an guarantee that you may maintain to have a have a look at, feature, and live well. Now who does now not want that?

Take some suggestions from the professionals!

If you are greater inspired to get your self began out with education for Brain Fitness, you can moreover want to recognize what the specialists take into account it. The following suggestions will permit you to gather Brain Fitness to the fullest:

Tip #01: Do you adore darkish chocolates? Here's every other reason to love them even extra. Dark chocolates produce dopamine it truely is essential in stylish brainwork. Chocolates are also rich in flavanols this is an antioxidant that lets in improve ordinary reminiscence.

Tip #02: Learn to play the guitar or piano. If you have got been planning to perform that however couldn't discover the time, this tip need to inspire you to prevent procrastinating. Learning the manner to play any musical tool makes you operate outstanding dimensions of your brain feature that is essential to preserving it in its satisfactory form.

Tip #03: Go and notice the Louvre (or every other museum). Another workout tip for thoughts fitness is going to an area and seeking to take in as lots records as you may. You can then write down a precis of what you have got placed out and understood for the duration of the day. This exercise allows your mind plasticity live at a wholesome diploma.

Tip #04: Try juggling a ball – not actually because of the fact it's miles fun or thrilling. It is also mentally hard. Throwing the ball and catching it allows sensory-guided movements to be finished. This also tests your eye-hand coordination in addition to your mind tactility.

Tip #05: Challenge the opposite hand. This may additionally moreover additionally sound like a real assignment, but is notably viable consistent with professionals. If you are proper surpassed, then workout doing certain sports with the left including brushing your enamel, consuming, and so forth. Doing this workout, you're specifically disturbing a whole new getting to know context out of your mind. This will then 'compel' the opportunity factor of the mind which does fewer sports activities.

Tip #07: Try Boogie, Tango, or Rumba. If you're down with attempting some thing extra amusing and physical tough, you can select to peer a dance teacher. Learning new moves and sweating it out are genuine sports activities that stability your thoughts and frame skills. Physical sports pump greater oxygen to the mind which allows masses in retaining the thoughts cells healthful.

Whether you are taking transport of as actual with inside the idea of Brain Fitness or no longer, you cannot cut fee the truth that your thoughts is in fact as vital as another organ and device for your body. Without any fragment of doubt, right care and nourishment are each important.

Chapter 6: The Power Of Brain Training

Brain schooling is critical for our mind to get sharpened, so locate an area it truly is quiet, and be aware to it that you are by myself and can be undisturbed, it might be at a relaxing place wherein nature can calm your frame and thoughts. You also can do yoga, take a seat on the ground, or in a chair, or others choose to lie down on their all over again.

Do some deep breaths, enjoyable your complete body, permit air go together with the float freely and try no longer to do not forget a few component else, however be cautious no longer to go to sleep.

Exercises that you could do along with your mind:

1.Read a e-book, any ebook that hobbies you, depend how many phrases one paragraph has. Count them over again, without a doubt to make sure which you have counted effectively. After a few instances with one paragraph, try to growth it to two, then when you are cushty doing that, boom your load until you may depend a whole net page. Do the counting mentally using your eyes most effective, now not counting out loud or pointing at the phrases.

2.Try counting backwards, from 10 to one, growing through way of doing it a hundred to as a minimum one.

3.Counting backwards from 100 to as a minimum one, skipping three numbers, for instance, a hundred, ninety seven, 90 four and so forth.

four.Choose a phrase or a word and, repeat it for your mind for 5 minutes. When your mind can do more attempt to acquire ten minutes of uninterrupted attention.

5.Take any fruit like an apple, banana, orange or any fruit you need and conserving it for your hand. Examine the fruit's shape, flavor, scent, and the sensations you get at the equal time as touching it.

6.Same as massive variety 5, however this time in preference to searching on the fruit without a doubt visualize it, examine the fruit for 2 mins, then close to your eyes and have a study the fruit's form, taste, perfume, and the sensations you get with the aid of touching it even as your eyes are closed.

7.Watch any object with out thinking any phrases approximately it, it is probably a spoon, fork, or a tumbler.

eight.Draw a circle or a triangle or any form you want, and then coloration it with a coloration you need, keeping your hobby at the drawing without thinking about whatever else. Try no longer to stress your eyes.

9.Do the equal exercise as in range 8, but this time in region of searching at the drawing, visualize the drawing to your mind along side your eyes closed. If you forget about what the drawing seems like, open your eyes to observe the decide again, then as soon due to the fact the photo is settled try last your eyes once more to visualize the drawing.

10.Same as with workout big variety nine however this time visualize collectively with your eyes open.

11.Lastly strive for approximately five minutes, to simply be with none mind, both along with your eyes open, or maximum human beings would possibly likely do that with their eyes closed.

How is your mind feeling now?

We can say that our thoughts is the busiest a part of our frame; it requires sharpening on a each day foundation. Sharpening our brain calls for exercise and attention, like the entirety else in life does. We brush our enamel 3 times a day, eat at the least 3 times a day, workout on a every day basis, and so on. Even 10 minutes a day of hobby carrying sports will provide you with extremely good outcomes.

Can you reputation well on topics now?

If you're this kind of folks who assume that they will multi-undertaking, then I am telling you that era doesn't buy the multi-tasking hype. When you multitask, you do now not attention on one assignment, instead you bounce from one assignment or interest to 3 other. What you don't realize is that you aren't helping yourself, you're really prolonging the final contact of all of the duties involved.

How are you able to tell your mind is functioning well?

Vital procedures are disrupted if our mind receives too much or too little of what it desires. It can wreak havoc with our thoughts and emotions when subjects are out of sync in our mind. If we are lacking sleep, probabilities are our alternatives and mind will impair our capability to pay attention.

These techniques will assist maintain our mind healthy and balanced:

1.Get enough sleep – If we don't have sufficient sleep or don't get enough relaxation we genuinely don't feature as well mentally, emotionally, and bodily. Our mind desires rest and downtime.

2.Get transferring – Exercise frequently to be able to increase the go with the flow of blood inside the thoughts and maintains you more alert. Be energetic 30 to 60 mins an afternoon or maximum of the instances in every week to get your frame and mind once more into alignment.

3.Light up your life – Proper lighting allows our thoughts feature properly, herbal lighting is the quality, which eases fatigue and depression for max humans, however in case you are jogging with too much lighting fixtures, see to it that you cowl your eyes with protective system or solar sunglasses, take a break each 20 to half of-hour from publicity with computer structures.

four.Do no longer smoke, in case you are a smoker, make a plan to stop. .

5.Control sicknesses together with diabetes and excessive blood strain which may be chronic ailments.

6.Don't drink alcohol or drink moderately.

7.Once you find out which you have a trouble along aspect your vision or hearing see your medical doctor or healthcare organization for assist.

8.If you have melancholy, get treatment.

nine.Do sports activities sports that require your mind to research and art work like studying a ebook, play games, board video video video games, puzzles and plenty of others.

10.Listen to tune — studies suggests that track calms the thoughts.

eleven.Slow down — don't rush subjects, it's crucial which you definitely take a seat down lower back and try to see the entire photo clearly so you may be able to do the proper factor and make the extraordinary selections viable.

Chapter 7: What Is Brain Training And Why It Matters?

Even despite the fact that we spend our days seeking out strategies to eat more healthy and get greater exercising, the one detail that won't be as clean is that our frame moreover has wishes for mind fitness. It calls for the mind to be saved sharp and actively pushed to be higher.

The mind is each the use of it or destroying the frame. It way that it will go to pot if you do now not provide your mind the proper stimulation over the years. Once the thoughts hobby begins offevolved to turn out to be worse, you may begin to see the shortage of intellectual reminiscence, lack of recognition, and every so often Dementia or Alzheimer's.

There's hundreds you could do to boost your thoughts health in your normal. It could make a massive distinction on your stylish mind fitness only a few mins a day spent performing thoughts activities. Here are multiple strategies you can do this.

Learning a current talent will sharpen the intellect. We are extra involved and happier if our brains study a few element new. You can analyze a remote places language; you could discover ways to play chess or possibly to shade water. All those bodily video games are notable education for the thoughts.

Get up and skip! It's terrible in your thoughts to put spherical all day and be sedentary. You must go out and stress spherical. Walking is a wonderful choice, or possibly a amusing night time day trip. Whatever you pick out out, you recognize that there are fewer reminiscence lapses and mentally complete of lifestyles individuals who are energetic.

Eat meals from the heart. Like each extraordinary part of the body, meals is notably tormented by mind schooling. Meat, blueberries, avocados, pumpkin seeds, and spinach are the terrific brain foods you can consume. Many different meals assist the mind to integrate at least one or of those into your diet plan each day.

Challenge the thoughts. You can do plenty of sports to keep your mind healthy. It's one manner to play mind video video video games like chess, puzzles, and sudoku. Computer software program software programs are also particularly designed to offer mind fitness sports activities which is probably scientifically designed to enhance cognitive popular overall performance.

Have a pleasant chuckle. Research has set up that laughter turns on and alarms the thoughts. For hours, the have an effect on of a fantastic tight giggle will ramp up your wondering. So find time in your day to smile, steal a study a comic story blog, and preserve out with individuals who make you chortle.

All those additives will decorate the overall health of your thoughts. The greater you operate your thoughts, the more likely you may have a first rate memory, sharp cognizance, and the more speedy you'll be capable of remedy troubles.

How Passive and Active Brain Training Can Improve Your Brain

When it involves shaping your thoughts, mind education is the modern day "craze." As it happens, there was an growth in reading to enlarge cognitive processing as scientists have found that the neurons on your mind make new institutions (that is known as mind plasticity) with each exceptional. It changed into ground-breaking technology at the same time as this became positioned and tested, regardless of the truth that it can't seem that way.

The mother stated, "use it or lose it" on the equal time as you've got been more younger, and this time period refers in your thoughts. Surprisingly, you can make new associations on your mind through the usage of your thoughts in unique strategies, that is concept to lessen your risk of ailments collectively with Alzheimer's, and you may make your thoughts stronger. There are count on tanks at the manner to teach the thoughts-passive and active thoughts training. What's the distinction, and what is your mind doing with the ones?

People realized thoughts Training Methods Once this idea that you could educate your brain, a present day marketplace appeared in a single day. Organizations collectively with Luminosity have created a useful company model for thoughts schooling. Nevertheless, you may actively educate your thoughts, even simple puzzles that have been spherical forever (and are free). Such forms of troubles like puzzles from the jigsaw, Sudoku, and the each day crossword puzzle will assist the thoughts make such new connections through the years.

Active thoughts gaining knowledge of blessings Learning the thoughts always should bring about many notable mind changes. Such benefits include extra fine processing tempo, superior quick-term memory in every verbal and visual-area, and advanced running memory. If you phrase that every one of these results revolve round your quick-time period reminiscence, you could marvel why that is important to you, but it's miles. Your short-time period reminiscence is in truth as vital on your prolonged-time period memory (or perhaps extra so). There are such loads of additives to your short-term reminiscence; scientists are not precisely high quality the way you maintain memories, additionally even though they have got a extraordinary concept. Short-term reminiscence must be Improved essentially approach you could machine statistics quicker and hold it longer earlier than each sending it off on your lengthy-term reminiscence or simply dropping the wondering. Long-time period results encompass more massive interest, expanded creativeness, and stepped forward announcement.

Passive thoughts training much like lively schooling Using your thoughts would make your mind happier, smarter, more potent, and further sturdy. It sounds just like the manner to transport is energetic mind learning, however what about cognitive exercise? Why even recollect passive getting to know if you may get a majority of these first-rate benefits from immoderate education?

In the era and purchaser global, passive mind education is at the upward push. There has been evidence that there are numerous kinds of mind education that could function for you, however nice in case you continuously exercise your mind correctly over the long time. Although your quick-term reminiscence is frequently laid low with lively studying, passive training ought to have prolonged-term results to your thoughts.

Besides, you can experience worn-out or dizzy via active mind education. After all, you are strolling very hard to your mind. You lose interest if you address your muscle tissue. Function the thoughts, get tired, and regain time. Passive thoughts training takes advantage of the truth that your mind desires to respond to stimuli as correctly as feasible-it has already laid down neural pathways. This sounds counterintuitive, however if you make the effort to create new neural connections, your thoughts have to have more than one paths that you may flow down while you reply to a stimulus, that is a remarkable thing. Passive mind analyzing is documented through the use of schooling early enthusiasts no longer to reason highbrow fatigue and decrease any symptoms and signs and symptoms and signs of thoughts fog in some unspecified time in the future of the day.

It uses generation for audio and seen mind education. There are every short-term and lengthy-time period profits in passive thoughts training. An introduced plus is that over the years, quick-time period advantages may be of lengthy-term interest.

Note, this is a latest and growing difficulty of technological knowledge approximately schooling the thoughts-mind. Both of those sorts can help the thoughts, and if you need to increase your noggin, there are numerous extraordinary bodily sports you can do. A lot of research is being performed proper now to decide how we will higher our brains, mainly in brain issues prevention and intervention. Consider your self busy and maintain in thoughts your mind thinking in case you want to hold yourself sharp for many years to go back again. These are the primary components of both notion kinds, so hold the brain going!

Brain Training Exercises

Bet you concept mind drills meant some problem like memorizing the mobile phone listing of NYC?

Well, memorization equipment are available that is probably a part of your thoughts education sports. Still, mind schooling these days has a amazing deal more to do with neurogenesis and neuroplasticity, of the human mind's these days decided abilities.

No one realized until approximately 12-15 years in the past that we humans were developing new thoughts cells, the technique described through manner of way of the term neurogenesis.

Such new cells amplify every day even as we feature them to a hospitable surroundings, due to this we cope with what the specialists name the ideas of mind health.

Most of those experts say the contemporary neurons are migrating to the hippocampus, an important part of your thoughts's reminiscence-preserving circuitry.

Would you want an outline of the entire manner of mind education sporting activities?

Evans and Burghardt make it very easy to recognize the concepts of neurogenesis and neuroplasticity and the manner to determine out the thoughts.

The time period neuroplasticity, with the useful resource of the way, is the time period utilized by specialists to explain how the thoughts reorganizes itself, every so often in mins after studying something new.

That's accurate, and we do not want to wait till there can be a massive weight of latest records crushing the skull till a turning element is reached, and there may be a huge shift.

The thoughts reorganizes itself as we realize. Still, we can also moreover moreover need to revisit the education and remember to attend to the' getting-enough-sleep' thing of thoughts fitness due to the reality this is at the same time as memory consolidation takes place.

Okay, so what is the brain health foundation, and the way do I exercising it?

The foundations of thoughts training sports activities sports are physical exercising, meals in conjunction with antioxidants and omega-three fatty acids, the sleep, stress control, and revolutionary studying opinions listed above.

Perhaps the maximum important of the pillars is physical workout, in an effort to be lousy information for us for the sofa potatoes.

The right information, however, is that the diploma and frequency of bodily exercising wished for neurogenesis and neuroplasticity want no longer entail an Olympic education scheme or maybe club of a gym.

To maximize blood glide to the thoughts, we want if you want to generate deeper, quicker respiration for approximately 10 mins some instances an afternoon. The deeper, quicker breathing will come from taking walks more fast than you already do.

When taking note of a stimulating lecture in your iPod, physical exercise does no longer prevent you from becoming a member of a fitness center or working to be had as well.

But with device like an workout ball and a few 5-pound dumbbells, like those used by 89-year-antique Bill and82-3 hundred and sixty 5 days-vintage Pat to maintain themselves in situation for his or her worldwide adventure adventures, you can be exceptional at the bodily exercise pillar.

Nutrition may also, of direction, be a large part of your brain training sports activities, this means that you need to set the processed food aside and boom the end result and greens. Surprisingly, on your brain health regimen, there may be a big function for omega-3 fatty acid, which wants to be taken in by means of the use of the use of what you devour, due to the fact your body does no longer generate it very correctly.

According to Evans and Burghardt, about 70 percentage of our neuron membrane is product of omega-3 fatty acids, and if it is not replenished, those membranes end up susceptible, and neuron-to-neuron interplay is concealed.

Fish is the excellent supply of omega-3 fatty acids, however if you do now not like consuming or cooking fish, a supplement may be so as.

When defined above, sleep is an critical part of your thoughts education sports activities, and that is proper facts for optimum parents, however you need to bear in mind to provide enough REM sleep for your brain, because of this that complete nights of sleep.

Managing pressure can be very important for neurogenesis and neuroplasticity because too much and too ordinary publicity to strain hormones will kill the ones newly born neurons and suppress neuroplasticity inside the very last neurons.

Some humans don't assume they need to take care of stress extra than more than one instances every week, but I would probable say you want to attend to heartbeat pressure.

Is it now not viable to sound? Not really whilst you recognize a way to do biofeedback with coronary heart charge variability, which teaches the heart to grow to be regular while you engage in cue questioning and respiratory pattern.

A brilliant aspect impact of biofeedback coronary coronary heart price variability? This opens up the higher thoughts centers of belief. A stronger mind than a self-control by way of using rest? You're playing.

And the brand new studying experience pillar is the very last pillar of mind health.

The experts say that the most huge new gaining knowledge of experience for neurogenesis and neuroplasticity is the shape of precise analyzing experience we gather whilst gaining knowledge of a modern-day language or device.

Not sure approximately you, but I do now not have a bargain time to exercise a brand new language or a current device, so I'll attempt out some of the automatic mind health applications.

I like what the Effects report has to mention about the simplest mind carrying sports tool, and the PNAS art work is just as exciting approximately the effects of the twin n returned sports activities.

These are guides I can do on my computer, and I can also want to make it lots less complicated for such mind schooling sports than I can for Spanish training.

Feel the tingling of your mind? If you do the ones thoughts drills, it'll.

Chapter 8: How Workout Trains The Thoughts?

The thoughts is man's maximum splendid organ. But it ought to not be taken as a take into account of route. To maintain it up and going, simulation and exercise are its best fodder. It protects moreover toward cognitive decline similarly to growing mind feature. Findings tell us that the the use of of mind by myself, the range of dendritic branches linking thoughts cells will increase assuredly.

Why is exercising our brains so crucial?

In the jargon of the laymen, the brain is vulnerable to being atrophied and killed without exercise. The benefits are each quick-time period (advanced hobby and memory, continuous mental clarity, smooth idea, and coordination) and lengthy-time period (advent of a "brain buffer" that protects in opposition to Alzheimer's).

How does exercising state of affairs the thoughts?

fitness manager describes how exercise impacts a couple of worrying system net websites and offers pleasure chemical materials like serotonin and dopamine that make us experience comfortable, satisfied, and euphoric.

Some techniques to train the thoughts, make certain the sound always and operation improve its standard performance are listed underneath: have interaction the thoughts with extraordinary duties: undertaking your mind to have a look at new responsibilities, particularly those you haven't expert earlier than.

Eggs: getting prepared a cutting-edge-day dish, analyzing an application for software program software, shopping in a one-of-a-type grocery shop, playing a modern day laptop recreation.

To manage the pc mouse, far flung TV, brush your tooth, or dial the telephone, switch the hand you usually use.

You'll find out that on the preliminary diploma, you are very uncomfortable and awkward in handling it. But don't worry that you educate the mind to be versatile and prepare it to address new obligations.

Your Brain Travel Stimulates is an outstanding way to accumulate the brain. It as well worked for our forefathers, whose nomadic lifestyle supplied extraordinary opportunities to visit new locations, have a take a look at new things, and find out unknown statistics.

Neurobics is a totally precise of mind carrying activities the usage of in sudden methods your 5 emotional experience and bodily senses, inspire you to disenchanted your regular workouts. They assist your mind produce its vitamins to enhance, preserve, and increase thoughts cells.

In a each day venture, strive the usage of a couple of of your senses: eggs. Learn as you chunk, have a study on the equal time as you are taking observe of a lecture.

Physical exercising Did that your mind regularly blessings from physical hobby? It is essential because it affects the fee of creation of latest neurons in our brains. Excellent mind stimulators are the chance of taking walks for an hour or walking.

Write "Read, write, examine," says Case Western Reserve Medical School's Dr. Amir Soas in Cleveland. Don't simply restriction your reading to newspapers and magazines. At the identical time, try and take a look at sorts of books. Alternate, non-fiction fiction. Not first-rate will they assist beautify your vocabulary, but they'll also attraction for your modern and sensible aspects.

Strengthen your memory. Try to memorize the maximum often used telephone numbers.

Try to bear in thoughts and recapitulate statistics and statistics which you have amassed in an afternoon. If the need arises, this could help you to remember it later.

Try to take into account the each day morning headlines you're studying.

There are masses of programs accessible to your memory to help. The recommendation is "Brain Age" or "Big Brain Academy" for the Nintendo DS. Specifically, the ones games are made to enhance memory.

It's a bendy component to have a look at. Never divorce learning from your self. Try to study one or information each day. Make it a dependancy. Tell your self what you've got found for the day in advance than you doze off. Help your children, grandchildren, buddies, buddies with their topics, plan, and plenty of others. Remedy issues Many newspapers have each day new sudoku and crosswords. Try your hand on ebook-selling brainteasers, riddles, and various styles of puzzles. On the net, you could even rent a remarkable deliver. Try to clear up the ones problems. Those sharpen your ability to clear up problems. Play scrabble and storm for 15 minutes each day over the cube of the Rubik.

Select a sentence from a mag or newspaper and keep the usage of the same words to make another paragraph.

Practice as soon as feasible, connecting the bits of a jigsaw puzzle. Boost the time it takes to clear up it.

Logic is the art of reasoning— finding an ordered collection of disparate elements. When shopping, do no longer use a written listing. Alternatively, using don't forget aids, collectively with forming a entire phrase, or one which may be completed through way of the use of which consist of a selected vowel or consonant to the belongings you want to shop for from the primary letters of the terms. Alternatively, use a few component works for you.

Listen to the morning data at the radio or television. Jot down the main factors of the records you keep in mind at some stage in the day. Every day try to upload new terms on your vocabulary. Each time you finish a chapter in a ebook which you wrote, summarize it as in short as feasible. Do the identical at the same time as you end the complete e-book.

Moving your arms to boost the thoughts: physical sporting sports that use your fingertips are recorded to stimulate the mind, which include crocheting, knitting, playing the piano, and so on. A mind map shows that the nerve endings in your fingertips suit greater mind areas than some other body area, besides probably the tongue and lips.

Sing To Solve problems Sing about some aspect that you're walking on at the same time as you're on my own in your private home. This will relax the thoughts. If you sing, it's far much less tough to rhyme than while you're each talking or writing. This is due to the fact sample reputation is first-rate for the proper brain.

Ways to an Healthier Brain

You may additionally want to start mind training for quite some motives or revel in the thoughts is eroding in preference to doing some thing approximately it. In this submit, I'm going to expose you 3 procedures to do something wonderful about your mind!

Physical exercising, a super way of life, and Mental workout are these form of bureaucracy. These are massive topics, of path, so examine at once to offer an reason for and gather on them.

Mental exercising Has so-referred to as plasticity, like with almost any location of your lifestyles. You understand, for path, what your our our bodies will amplify even as you hold in shape enough. It is because you located a pressure on them, and they are going to answer to it via manner of growing, so it does not enjoy like plenty extra the following time you throw plenty strain on them.

It's plasticity. And it is also suitable on your coronary coronary heart. Need to be in primary school and have a look at the important ideas of mathematics? You have been vain at the start to do these x-something-like calculations because of the reality you by no means saw them earlier than. Yet you bought higher at multiplying figures after some training and exercise with them. And not simplest the figures with which you have practiced, all figures. You need to brief increase some issue if you have emerge as fast at it and decided out some pointers.

Then with some thing else in mind, it works the same manner. If you want a higher reminiscence, what better manner to use your memory greater regularly (region greater strain on it) than to use it in some of methods?

Research has established that you broaden extra' brain muscle' when you workout your mind frequently and in creative strategies. But then how are you to educate them? How are you' genuinely more likely to apply your memory?'

It has to do with precise behaviors that push your thoughts similarly to the development of your muscular tissues. These encompass: sports activities that make you have got were given had been given all of your senses and interact in new matters (subjects that test the thoughts in a manner you have not skilled earlier than) Activities like analyzing an tool and playing it, studying a contemporary language or painting permit you to use some imagination whilst managing more than one mind regions

Things you need to devise, along with chess or painting.

We often advocate doing a platform or video video games from time to time with families or pals and gaining knowledge of once in a while something new. That is probably a tool, or some component with paintings/format, or a simply one in every of a kind language, a few factor that you think is proper to analyze.

Physical workout Your universe is made up of nerve cells or neurons, and those muscular tissues for your body manage your frame with the useful aid of getting to feel and' measuring' the whole thing. They make connections for your thoughts and make certain that your frame's frightened device works nicely. So, while you growth extra muscle and practice any' actions,' your body desires more nerve cells, and your mind dreams more neurons to regulate it all.

So, you honestly should schooling consultation each day, each day of the week, for at minimal half-hour. It can be a few component this is pretty intimidating, as a minimum. It may additionally motive you to increase muscle, and it's going to additionally motive you to lose fats and therefore increase your brain.

But do no longer clearly sit down down each day in your mattress and carry out a little take a seat down-u.S.A.And carrying activities for 1/2-hour. It's correct in your mind to move outside and do a real endeavor!

For example, in case you'd circulate playing basketball, you may research what to learn how to shoot, what to jump better, how to dribble quick, perhaps a few basketball hints. These are all competencies that require an entire lot of schooling to perform for your frame and thoughts, and you've got got were given a more potent thoughts even as you draw close those!

Good manner of existence The 1/3 issue that regulates your thoughts is in all likelihood the maximum important. A incredible life-style. This manner: the second purpose is that one of a kind humans despite the fact that encourage you. Okay, in case you're no longer jealous. If you're, I actually have to mention: do not be. Other people may have terrific perspectives of factors, various things about which they understand hundreds, unique perspectives of specific subjects. And in case you be aware of them and speak to them approximately issues, you will get hundreds of recommendations and belief for topics. Because what is a better motivation and thought than, as an example, some human beings apprehend you may design matters and ask you to create a brand for them?

Eating nicely: in case you don't eat sufficient, you don't have enough muscle, mind, or strength to be concerned and deliver interest to subjects/wondering.

When you consume an excessive amount of, maximum of your thoughts may be complete of body-controlled neurons (but overeating is commonly better than consuming too little). Make positive you have got were given breakfast, drink sufficient, and eat a number of different things (the secret's range).

Sleeping nicely: similar to ingesting, in case you're now not sleeping nicely, you do now not have the strength to prepare and consciousness on yourself. Very younger kids require 11-13 hours of sleep, which will become less and plenty an awful lot less at the identical time as you turn out to be older. When someone reaches young adults (high college), they want at the least 9 hours of sleep. But the quandary proper right here is that nature goals young adults to live up past due while college makes them awaken early. You want a exceptional deal less sleep whilst you're older (25+), spherical 6-7 hours a night time. BUT, how a whole lot sleep you need relies upon on how a good deal you're doing in sooner or later. Do now not have a look at those numbers exactly, and the frame is aware of how a good buy it desires to sleep.

Being busy: some thing that works is foremost an lively lifestyles if correctly finished, nearly as right as mind training gamers. If you are not stimulated to look at stuff or do new subjects each day, your brain might not amplify. And it is easy if you have the stress. But it isn't commonly easy for anybody to get the foundation. You get the electricity to be assured, brave, and to have human beings spherical you.

Being social: and why it is so crucial to have people round you is because it's crucial to be social. This is because of the truth we people have this kind of complicated mind due to the truth we are very social animals. We want that mind to hold tune of all of the human beings we apprehend, to preserve tune of a verbal exchange or discussion, almost all we do is social in everyday life. So the extra you speak to human beings, do matters with humans, play a group game, and so forth, the more your thoughts grows.

The second cause is that unique human beings regardless of the reality that inspire you. Okay, if you're now not jealous. I actually have one problem to mention if you are: do no longer be. Many humans can also have unique perspectives of factors, one in every of a type thoughts approximately which they recognise masses, unique perspectives of precise topics. And in case you pay attention to them and communicate to them about matters, you may get plenty of suggestions and concept for subjects. Because what's a higher motivation and idea than, as an instance, a few people understand you can layout topics and ask you to create a logo for them?

Exercise, New Brain Cells and Depression

Aerobic exercise, a far flung and unpleasant memory in most North American circles, has reared its unsightly head all all over again. Don't decorate your hopes, and I may not endorse that aerobic workout is not that specific for us, in the end. In truth, robust new generation tells us that there are a number of greater correct reasons to include aerobic workout into our lifestyles plan.

Deterioration of the mind and deterioration in cognition are taken into consideration commonplace competencies of getting older. Nonetheless, it changed into obvious that not in truth clearly every body is going down this slippery slope on the identical pace or to the same diploma. Individual variations inside the common overall performance of highbrow and brain function in antique age indicate that impairment and regression do no longer have an impact on anybody, nor do they inherently need to be getting older characteristics.

Because of this widespread locating and the growing getting older population in many countries spherical the arena, there can be a developing hobby in evaluating the opportunity that venture or enhancing positive behaviors must prevent or opposite the cognitive and neural decline in older adults.

In truth, new mind cells can be created, new blood assets to feed them, and the harm carried out may be reversed. The aerobic exercising is a hero in the sport. The different is the reminiscence studying that works.

There come to be plenty of discussion approximately the realistic nature of growing new brain cells (man or woman neurogenesis), so an vital aim has been to evaluate their impact on living people, away from experimental models and non-human experimenters.

The preliminary aerobics experiments and their capacity to supply new mind cells and a sparkling deliver of brain blood to feed them were performed on mice. It grow to be confirmed exactly in which aerobic exercising stimulated the blood amount inside the brain and whether this modified into coupled with the ensuing neurogenesis. Yoga has been established to have a powerful impact on an uncommon vicinity known as the dentate gyrus, a hippocampal sub-place, among all mind areas. This is the only sub-location that allows the growth of new person mind cells.

Besides, the exercising-caused upward thrust in dental gyrus blood quantity grow to be related exactly with put up mortem increase measures of latest thoughts cells. For the mice, a lot.

Next, within the same hippocampal education of exercising humans, maps of thoughts blood volume have been generated through the years the usage of comparable MRI technology on human topics. As in mice, exercise emerge as shown to have a number one effect on the blood quantity of the dentate gyrus, and those upgrades have been discovered to correlate exactly with cardiopulmonary and cognitive function. Taken together, those consequences recommend that there can be nevertheless an unique correlation amongst wealth dental gyrus blood extent and exercise-triggered neurogenesis. That exercise is differentially directed at dental gyrus, an area vitally vital for reminiscence and worried in cognitive ageing. The backside line is, at the equal time as you exercising aerobically, you may improve your mind.

Otherwise, human beings of any age regularly go through dwindled deductive capacity in some of thoughts areas, accompanied by manner of way of degradation and bargain of thoughts tissue.

Concentration, and working reminiscence exams. These improvements are accompanied with the beneficial useful resource of altered measurements of mind interest and an boom in the quantity of mind tissue that translates into greater effective every day sharpness.

We all recognize that cardio exercising makes us feel right as an entire lot as we avoid it. But we don't all experience accurate all the time, unfortunately.

Every yr, 18.Eight million over 18-yr-antique North Americans are crushed by way of way of way of conceitedness that creates a depression that can not be willed or disregarded. Depression impacts anyone regardless of age, area, or social popularity. Persistence of terrible temper may be characterized as big melancholy beyond the period of the initial lousy occasion or strain.

It has best been installation in the remaining ten years that there have been new baby neurons within the adult mind. These infant brain cells appear to be vital to discover diffused changes in the environment and to link feelings to the out of doors context.

This style has evolved the idea that disrupted the boom of new thoughts cells is a motive of depression, and stimulation of latest infant neurons is critical for a fulfillment antidepressant motion.

Recent paintings, in addition to assessing man or woman differential factors, demonstrates that intellectual and brain degradation isn't always unchangeable and that the older grownup mind continues some plasticity that can be used to contrary deterioration and decline, which can also additionally already be going on and otherwise prevent it.

Valid virtual going for walks reminiscence learning addresses the proper mind function, which proves essential to any active mental method if dedicated to the science that substantiates it. Whether you're analyzing, writing, talking, listening, fixing troubles, playing an tool, or simply simple thinking, your running reminiscence frames the motion for you.

When your thoughts grows older, your mind can broaden sharper and stronger, and pc-based totally completely education systems prove to be the way to make it take vicinity.

Now is the time to build up resources to your mind. Increasing the vital highbrow functionality of operating reminiscence, recognition, and interest is in no way too overdue.

So, it is not approximately "the usage of it and dropping it," it's miles approximately studying it and making extra of it.

Chapter 9: Good Habits For The Brain

You've heard it before, I'm sure: the mind is sort of a muscle. So the stronger it gets, the greater you operate it. They will wither and die if your brain cells (neurons) are not used. You can assemble a suitable buffer, however, and enlarge new roads. What found are carrying sports activities you can do in your lifetime, as a way to offer your thoughts a extremely good exercising, maintain it easy, and beautify your thoughts in a few times. These behavior are going to do you tremendous right now and hopefully pay off in the future as they'll help prevent Alzheimer's and dementia's sickness.

1 Practice pleasant thinking Tell yourself that you are going to get through them if awful topics take place to your existence. Know that you have the energy to obtain this and that they will not final all the time. On the alternative hand, revel in the

extraordinary matters that come your manner. Seek to appearance the fantastic in the global and exquisite humans as you go through your day. New pathways are original within the mind via questioning this way. Yes, the thoughts can change, and it is known as neuroplasticity. Your brain has built extraordinarily-modern, notable pathways through cultivating a incredible attitude. How specific is it? Besides, research at New York University showed that it stimulated the rostral anterior cingulate and the amygdala whilst humans engaged in excessive nice questioning. Both parts of the brain are every suffering from emotional responses and anxiety, as well. Therefore, your emotional reactions can be progressed by manner of way of moving into a incredible dependancy, and you can reduce your threat of affected by despair.

It is believed that effective mind can launch serotonin, a mind chemical that makes you feel excellent, is the remaining motive to steer you to be wonderful. And, because of the preliminary satisfied thoughts you had, you turn out to be feeling even better.

2 Engage in everyday exercise There are such some of benefits in your mental and physical health, and studies keeps to find out increasingly more motives to training session. There are excellent advantages for your mind, and I actually have blanketed some of the highlights underneath.

Current evolutionary theories say that we're extra sensible because of physical hobby. After their prey (power walking), earliest ancestors will jog, and anthropologists advise this caused human mind development. Research indicates superior memory average overall performance after strolling individuals. Also, a 2007 take a look at through Columbia University placed that going for walks out 4 times in line with week resulted in progressed production of neurons within the dentate gyrus, an area that is vital to reminiscence.

Exercising gives to the mind and notes that for a few hours after exercise, you may see a sharpening on your interest inside the brief term. Perhaps if you're suffering to concentrate at artwork, the morning could be a first-rate time to exercising. It can prevent Alzheimer's ailment in the long run.

It has been tested that exercising decreases high blood pressure. If you have got have been given excessive blood pressure, there may be an improved threat of a thoughts hemorrhage, which can result in long-time period thoughts harm.

A style of neurotransmitters, along with endorphins, serotonin, dopamine, and norepinephrine, are released into the mind even as you exercising. These are healthy mood boosters that reduce your risk of depression.

Exercise in older women decreased cognitive decline. The blessings had been confirmed to girls who walked most effective 90 mins every week of their 70s and 80s. The extra concerned the person became, however, the better the advantages. It is idea that workout can decorate neural fibers, synapses, and capillaries. In cognitive tests, older those who strolled did no longer perform in addition to folks that walked faster. Someone who took greater than 17 seconds to stroll 50 ft is an indication of a sluggish stroll. For later benefits, preserve up your strolling regime now.

It's clean that on the same time as you workout, there are each short-term and long-term blessings to your thoughts fitness. To maintain your thoughts solid, try and revel in what you're doing and mix matters up a piece bit.

three Go dancing. There's masses to consider at the same time as you dance. You need to make quick alternatives, be alert, preserve in mind the motions, have in mind of your companion, preserve music of your frame in location, and keep up a correspondence with the song's tempo. It's no surprise to take a look at that dance stimulates numerous specific additives of the mind-giving an effective workout to both the thoughts and body. As you dance, the cerebral cortex and hippocampus can be used, and dancing might require complex neural pathways. The thoughts is growing larger and more potent and more privy to cognitive problems in later lifestyles via the improvement of those new pathways.

A test from the New England Journal of Medicine in evaluation numerous entertainment sports activities that helped to reduce the risk of dementia. Those who danced often had a reduced threat of dementia of seventy six percentage. This decreased hazard, each useful behaviors, became greater tremendous than studying or doing crossword puzzles.

4 Eat healthily and not too much to maintain a balanced weight-reduction plan high in whole grains, end end result, and vegetables for better bodily and highbrow health. Many merchandise, however, are suitable for the brain. These consist of end quit result, vegetables, and proteins, which includes eggs, soy, peas, nuts, and seeds. For assist defend in the direction of Alzheimer's sickness, cinnamon, rosemary, turmeric, basil is all taken into

consideration. Drinking fruit or vegetable juice can help shield mind cellular damage as it consists of excessive levels of antioxidant polyphenols. People who drink these juices are lots a great deal much less susceptible to developing Alzheimer's infection. Of course, the ones people may moreover have had an regular wholesome manner of existence, so it is now not pretty much the food.

five Off the Television, Watching an excessive amount of television can also additionally boom your danger of growing Alzheimer's. For each greater hour, an afternoon spent looking tv, the threat improved through 1.Three percent. The extra hours spent inside the the the front of the tv manner much less time available for unique obligations a very good way to deliver your thoughts a very good workout, not only is television viewing a passive pastime.

6 Play video video video games If you want to sit down down within the the front of the TV, you can be involved at the identical time as you're at the Couch. The reaction anticipate it is video video games or now not. Obviously, in balance. Researchers discover that playing video video video video games is good for the mind. Research performed with the resource of Bavelier has tested that gamers are more concentrated than non-game enthusiasts and can track records. Brain scans positioned that the brains of gamers have been more effective and quicker on the same time as paying hobby (they may tune six gadgets straight away. The commonplace is 4). Many works have demonstrated that gamers are greater progressive, higher preference-makers, advanced visible abilities, and higher coordination of the hand-eye. Now, as a partner of COD, can I inform this to my husband?

7 Puzzles and video games Depending on the type, puzzles, and games prompt considered one of a kind parts of the mind. Engage in some thing which can make you accept as true with you studied. Play chess, puzzles of right judgment, anagrams, video video video games of technique, crosswords, sudoku, mahjong, jigsaws, card video video games, scrabble. Try to exercise severa particular areas of your mind and boom the issue even as it becomes too dull.

Bunge and Mackey had board, card, and video video video games finished through college college students, which confused both their price of wondering or their ability to motive. After 8 weeks, the wondering capability licensed college university students observed their non-verbal comprehension rankings upward push by using using 32 elements. The tempo of certified processing college students noticed a 27% development in their regular general overall performance ratings.

eight Discover new topics. You collect new connections between neurons and current ones while you examine a few component new. It's no longer pretty a good deal taking guides or increasing your information in new regions that you have a study new matters. It's approximately adjusting to each day adjustments. For instance, you'll probable complain approximately the difference in case your personal laptop or social media app gets an update. For a moment, but, recall your mind. It's used to the antique manner of strolling, and the code does not ought to paintings very hard. The alternate technique that you want to expect consciously once more, which leads to new paths being original. You've given a workout to your mind. So, the subsequent time you find your self facing a mission, in location of giving up, commit to conquering it. You will not exceptional enjoy a feel of success, but your brain also can be larger!

9 Don't see intelligence as a static problem. Studies with the useful resource of Dweck and associates determined that after college college students are advocated to apprehend that the mind develops new connections and evolves grade by grade via studying, their math grades extended. It is easy to assume as adults that we are all whole in our expertise and improvement. You're each accurate at a few factor right now, otherwise you are not. I preference this bankruptcy shows that your mind will hold growing, and the more you have got were given, the more pathways. Shake off any labels which you get as a infant. Give matters a skip, attempt to study a ultra-

modern capability, or face the heel of Achilles. If you've got were given determined on to paintings in your Achilles heel, have a look at that there may be a couple of way to examine some thing in case you're suffering. Take a current course for yourself.

10 Read a e-book Once you compromise all of the manner all the way all the way down to the particularly soothing studying challenge, there may be lots involved. Your mind is kept busy as you need to save data approximately what you have located and been able to get it via the ebook as you enhance. Who end up stated about that individual one hundred pages in the past? As you supply the trends defined in phrases to lifestyles in your thoughts, you furthermore may prompt your creativity and creativeness. That's fiction. There is also the opportunity to take a look at new regions you do not realize approximately

by way of way of manner of exploring the non-fiction phase. If you are a loose kindle ebook collector, make certain you're placing apart time to look at them.

It furthermore appears how ingesting too frequently can purpose thoughts changes. Eating too many excessive-calorie factors (people with lots of fat and sugar) may also want to exchange the mind, making it more likely to over-eat a human. Change is much like what takes location even as a drug addict will become someone. Another research has tested that overeating can decorate the risk of reminiscence loss for an character. People over 70 who consume spherical 2143 and 6000 calories consistent with week were appreciably much more likely to have excessive blood strain as folks who ate up about six hundred and 1525 energy an afternoon. The danger to individuals who ate masses much less than 2143 strength an afternoon turn out to be no longer obvious. It is theorized that overeating induces modifications within the brain that delivered on troubles with memory.. Change is just like what takes location whilst a drug addict will become a person. Another studies has verified that overeating can boom the risk of reminiscence loss for an man or woman. People over 70 who devour round 2143 and 6000 strength every week were extensively more likely to have hypertension as people who fed on approximately six hundred and 1525 strength a day. The danger to folks that ate lots less than 2143 energy a day changed into now not obtrusive. It is theorized that overeating induces modifications inside the thoughts that brought approximately problems with memory.

Bench Press for Your Brain

We all recognise what's occurring to our body because it grows older.

Without interference (an Activity/exercising software program application), we understand that our muscle companies are losing, our lung capacity is lowering, our heart is becoming weaker, our bones have end up fragile, our flexibility and mobility are falling, our reaction time is slowing, our posture is slowing down. We are becoming more vulnerable to disorder and damage.

Unless, of course, we stay a glaringly lively way of existence (one in which we spend severa energy regularly, go with the flow, convey, pressure our body... Doing subjects physically constantly).

I spoke in advance on this net internet site on-line about the idea of biological age (furthermore known as physiological age), and we have showed that via the use of the use of regulating first-rate variables (eating regimen, life-style, exercise, strain tiers), we are in a position to turn our frame clock decrease back absolutely. Although we may be fifty (chronologically), we may be capable of' collect' the body same to that of a everyday thirty-12 months-vintage (in terms of cardiovascular feature, staying strength, bone density, blood stress, flexibility).

If you have were given have been given been punishing your body for fifty years, it may, of route, be a special tale... But at the least you could step by step turn the clock again and see a huge improvement in vitamins, bodily function, and ordinary health.

With a huge percentage of the populace, what takes place (usually) is that we get to a point in time whilst we save you shifting as masses. We do not increase, stroll, hammer, climb, easy, work... Do bodily topics. And our body starts offevolved offevolved to age at a faster charge as speedy as this takes area. It is difficult to quantify (the developing vintage fee) as it varies from person to character... But truly permit's go along with it... The fee is a whole lot higher.

(Including our successful opposite numbers).

Retirement need to be referred to as the-beginning-of - the-give up for loads humans; they surrender doing pretty a good deal all that stored them in shape (I'm thinking about it from a health and paintings mind-set right here... Now not from a extraordinary attitude).

I don't assume we are all hired until we're 90 five... But the day they surrender for some human beings is the day they begin the usage of their minds and our our bodies (in a enormous manner).

They begin to go to pot the day.

Interestingly, on the equal time as you recollect that day, how satisfied many humans are.

And at the identical time as it's far commonplace and' everyday' for a number of us to teach our our our our bodies at the way to live physical extra youthful, relatively, most people do now not consciously take a comparable approach in terms of retaining our mind in shape (i.E., consciously' exercising' our thoughts as we do our our our our bodies).

Exciting, at the same time as we have a look at these statistics:

1) People usually mentally sluggish down as they age... Short-time period memory loss (wherein may be my keys?), slower processing of records, locating it extra hard to consciousness and pay interest, becoming much less complex to confuse,

being pressured, and appearing to be plenty less progressive and plenty less adventurous.

2) They're no longer imagined to! Multiple research (and subjective opinion) say that our thoughts, like each different muscle (nicely, it is now not a muscle, but you get my issue), wants to learn how to live in shape. Except for humans with particular medical situations, we find out that humans who've stayed mentally energetic as they age commonly enjoy minimal (or no) decline of their mind function level.

The 2d we cease to use it... We are beginning to lose it.

The correct information is that our mind (like our frame) is exceptional and might adapt at any age. We can (to a few diploma) contrary a number of the harm (if no longer most).

It's accurate to be physically in form, however what if we've got were given a mind like a Dalmatian? What's the aspect of having four percent body-fats, Olympian biceps and muscle corporations on our legs?

So proper here are my suggestions for developing and preserving a excessive-regularly occurring usual performance mind after hundred years of assisting humans get bodily in form.

1. Set the desires.

The 2d we prevent placing goals is on the same time as we begin to pass backward. We do not need to expect, plan, rationalize, treatment, or create issues without desires (a lot).

2. Smile, Laugh.

Laughing, being dumb, and having amusing even as your age is not illegal.

Even even though a few grumpy vintage farts are going to take me on this mission... They're wrong.

"Hey, Johnnie... Pull my finger."

three. Game.

"We may want to now not preserve playing because of the fact we amplify vintage. We grow antique because of the fact we prevent playing. "Good human beings inside the global are a (nearly) 70-12 months-vintage couple skiing, the usage of mountain bikes, strolling up and down dunes, walking, lifting weights, travelling, assisting others, playing sensible jokes, and placing out with' stupid' children.

4. Study.

You do not need to get your Ph.D. Back to college. (Perhaps) But likely talk brief publications, seminars... Something to blast the cerebral cobwebs out and make the rusty cogs flip again.

Once they give up faculty, maximum people (consciously) prevent gaining knowledge of.

One of my (Rona) group is fifty . Last 12 months she (for the first time) began university. When she is sixty-four, she can graduate collectively with her bachelor's degree (in Exercise Science) and has already knowledgeable me that she can hold to take a look at as quick as she completes her modern-day path. She said to me the alternative day. "It's the outstanding I ever did... In my existence!" (Condolences to her husband!).

five. Learn a ultra-modern language.

Evidence tells us that people who communicate (regularly) languages mature (mentally) at a slower price than their unilingual (made up... I assume) friends. We stay (mentally) in shape for longer... It even slows Alzheimer's onset.

So, if three languages had been spoken...

6. Creatively painting yourself.

Something to study... Start your blog, a ebook, a few poetry, a business plan.

Painting, portray, sculpting... My father started out out to shade at sixty five. And he is a great professional artist now.

Something invented... Crusty older men are the various finest inventors... You crusty antique guys, come on... Invent it! Invent a few element!

7. Write. Read.

And now not simply romantic novels... Read belongings you are the usage of your thoughts... You are a hint frustrating. Note, motive, make you consider you studied; exercising your thoughts.

8. Seek deliberately to endure in mind subjects.

There it's far. All you want is to dust it off.

Find photos of your antique school and contact all of your classmates.

Try and don't forget moments in time (and revisit them on your thoughts).

The next-door buddies of your first husband, the brothers... Name (you kissed one).

nine. Do a few exercising exercises of the thoughts.

Crosswords-a laugh to your thoughts and celebrated for it.

Puzzles, you recognize... Troubleshooting matters... Force your self to calculate, motive, purpose.

The terrific time for mind-education is when you have time on your arms... In the auto, bus, ready rooms on the train. Do problems with math, spell words, attempt to bear in mind precise records... Hmm, what is the DNA all over again?

What's Poland's capital?

10. That's incorrect. Have a plan.

To maintain you busy, to talk, to prepare, to remedy problems, to maintain in thoughts... Overall, the mind's bench pressing.

Starting a non-profits employer, developing a small business enterprise company, restoring your' fifty six Buick, scaling Everest... Anything that keeps you stimulated, gaining knowledge of, adapting, developing, and in form, mentally.

Now, what modified into the favourite coloration of my first lady pal, and what changed into the perfume she'd constantly been wearing?

Hang on for one minute... What changed into the decision of her!!

Build a Better Brain

In a manner, the mind is much like a toddler, and as a mom, you are on pinnacle of factors of its increase and nicely-being. Many human beings do this nicely, on the equal time as others do it appreciably, as is the case with maximum parents. Because the mind is so healthful, shifting away from the wheel and cruising on automobile-pilot through life is sometimes easy, however doing so is doing your self an injustice. History shows that in all chance the human species has created a number of top notch people and that most of them are of their personal making. Each of our minds has plenty capacity-probably extra than you may accept as true with, and ultimately, you and most effective you could unencumber yours. It's now not clean, however it is well worth it; why not make the maximum of it with one life to stay?

There are techniques on the way to change your thoughts and artwork your manner to a higher life. Now, there are a selection of things you may do to improve the mind, and everybody wants to take diverse steps relying on who they are or what they do, so the list is handiest a outstanding guiding principle. You are on the proper tune in case you're already doing an entire lot of these objects, and you're privy to it. If no longer, try them, and I can pretty a good deal assure that with a extra appreciation of life, they may make you mentally more difficult.

Rest-Sleep sufficient in no precise order. Insufficient sleep has a massive impact on temper and performance. The foundation for quite some the ones different steps is to have a properly-fed and nicely-rested thoughts; without this, you could not have strength for extra else.

Meditate-Talk to someone who constantly does this, and they'll praise their blessings. Explore meditation with a neuroscientist and they will reveal that it has a profound effect on the thoughts and the ability to alternate the brain's bodily form. Of example, meditation is the most conclusive proof which you have the strength to control your thoughts consciously. Unfortunately, the pointers in this list can also be the hardest and maximum time-eating, however properly properly honestly really worth it.

Exercise & Diet — You already apprehend you will try this for genuine bodily situation, however it's also very critical to your highbrow fitness; do no longer underestimate the price of blood flowing into your mind. Get this coronary coronary heart pumping spherical your apartment thru taking a swim, dancing or leaping rope. Take breaks for a brisk walk or some yoga from your day. Remove sugars and ingredients which might be subtle. Eat hundreds of fruit, vegetables and nuts, but now not too much; over-eating will virtually take a few bounces out of your stroll.

Music / Art-Take a seat at the piano or drum set if you do now not play song. If you do no longer have a paintbrush or clay, pick it. Even despite the fact that you are licking. All you do is do it. It's amusing and suitable for you. When you hesitate to play an tool, sing or dance at least. If you're no longer willing to the conventional arts, take a few innovative pictures or mess around in Photoshop as a minimum.

Language-Yes, you're well past the sensitive time to have a take a look at a modern-day language. Most probable you're in no manner going for you to make or pay attention all of the sounds wanted for fluency. Nonetheless, do no longer bear in mind it. Learning a ultra-modern language is a outstanding mental exercising and can be very beneficial in making pals, journeying and operating. And I'm going to extend that to encompass programming languages which might be moreover useful, tough and a laugh.

Hobbies-There are many benefits to choosing up a cutting-edge interest or gaining knowledge of a ultra-modern craft. Quilting allows decorate imagination and excellent motor abilties. Fly-fishing is likewise improving your motor abilties and getting you out, surrounded via manner of nature. Birding extends your memory, every visible and auditory. Your capability to prepare, prepare and join works through the use of the use of training a recreation. Practically any new activity that you choose out up will give you extensive mission and pleasure.

Play Brain Games-Games have splendid capability to sharpen your mind as they may be superb-tuned to a specific assignment and difficult sufficient to hold you focused on it. With the appearance of on line mind health applications, you may now exercise in one handy region your reminiscence, verbal functionality, consciousness, hassle-fixing, visuospatial functionality, and more.

Coordination / Balance / Engine Skill workout— Play with balls, be it juggling, ping pong, or a entice endeavor. Know the manner to tie the knots. Practice status on one leg or strolling like gadgets alongside a balancing beam (better yet, doing yoga or dancing). Play a Jenga interest or

Operation sport. Try balancing items on or in opposition to your neck, hands, or toes. These can also sound like kid's video games, but there may be a motive why kids do them: they're interesting, and they'll be splendid for you!

Join A Club-It's like a present day interest, however with a social twist. It's a fact that socialization and culture make you happier and more healthy. Join a set of writers, a sports sports membership, a softball group, or PTA. Volunteering is also suitable, as it has all the advantages of a club with the brought benefit of creating a distinction within the lives of others.

Memorize Everything-Start small and flow as a good deal as bigger, extra complicated topics. Try a track, a poem, a fave film conversation or a well-known speak. For no different useful cause than to stretch your mind, take a look at PI to 30 digits.

Read approximately all African countries- and then their capitols.

Jigsaw Puzzles & Model Building-Find an area to artwork on a jigsaw puzzle or assemble a model slowly in your own home. It's a great way to exercising your experience of area and a relaxing destroy from existence. If you cannot find out that unique piece, simply do not get too disenchanted!

Write-It want to be if writing isn't always a every day part of your lifestyles. And I'm not thinking about emails from businesses. Do some factor that is imaginitive and verbal. Start a weblog, hold a diary, write a poem, or discover a penpal.

Breathe & Relax-Stress is a killer of the thoughts. If you are too involved, you have were given were given to discover a way to loosen up. Start with the useful resource of the use of taking deep, calming breaths and then circulate on from there, whether or no longer it is a ebook porch, a kayak pond, a garden collectively along with your plants, or a few aspect else that makes you sense cushty.

Overcome a Weakness / Challenge Yourself-You mentally red meat up the perception which you have the energy over your life whenever you positioned a purpose and achieve it. It makes you revel in strong, willing and organized for the following challenge higher. It reminds you of your thoughts and life's exquisite capability.

Note, you're making lifestyles out of it-cliché, but very real. In your head, certainly, the perception is constructed up, and a sturdy, activated thoughts is much more likely to construct a excellent, fun international view. Don't get wrapped up in what you can't do or what you are not-the ones are commonly all falsehoods and excuses. Each people has a gem inside us, waiting to be mined; start exploring in and you could find out factors of you which you have ignored or in no way diagnosed for a long time. There is room for improvement constantly-no character has ever hit the restrict.

Chapter 10: Feed Your Brain - Keep Your Mind

We have been selling a healthy way of lifestyles's position in retaining thoughts fitness for a while now. Another new test offers similarly proof, however we figured we need to focus on some practical issues as to why that is so in advance than we get into it.

A sincere concept that doesn't require a Ph.D. Is that any organ for your frame, which encompass your brain, needs a healthful supply of blood to get right of entry to nutrients and oxygen. This is one motive why coronary coronary heart disorder is so regularly connected with intellectual health problems, including dementia. You must no longer be surprised in case your foot stops operating nicely in case you positioned a tourniquet round your arm to reduce off the blood supply.

It's the identical in your eyes. When you keep doing things which may be terrible in your cardiovascular device, which includes sitting spherical and eating chips all day prolonged, your coronary order will sooner or later have a disaster, and this isn't always proper data on your mind. Your mind uses about 20% of the oxygen you breathe and the energy you consume. Your coronary heart muscle is responsible for getting matters to the proper area to avoid your thoughts from on foot correctly.

The benefits of lifelong learning are widely known, and the thoughts is constantly challenged to maintain it easy. But if you do not integrate that attempt with doing what is wanted to preserve your neurovascular machine wholesome, you can't sincerely realize the benefit. You may also have test loads approximately neurogenesis and synaptogenesis, which is your brain's daily re-connection, which takes place on the same time as you stay mentally lively and helps maintain your thoughts agile. However, this method may additionally need to best perform properly if blood vessels near all this reengineering are nutritious sufficient to be doing their pastime. Otherwise, wherein is the gasoline, vitamins, and oxygen required to reshape the paintings?

Believe of neurogenesis as an reasonably-priced housing improvement becoming a member of an modern-day network and the roads because of the truth the deliver of blood to assist the houses. If you have been the developer building this new improvement, in case you did no longer attend the modern-day methods first, you will no longer get very some distance. Not pleasant are the roads required to get in and out in their houses for the state-of-the-art owners, however they may be had to transport all of the timber and cement for the numerous people to are to be had and construct the brand new houses, and do away with all the garbage. Likewise, to artwork effectively, new thoughts cells and new thoughts cellular connections require stable roads (neurovascular tool).

In conjunction with this, a modern day sizable review, quality launched this month, estimates that 33% of the threat of dementia is because of infection of small blood vessels inside the mind. Three thousand 4 hundred males and females over the age of sixty 5 participated on this 12-twelve months test for occasional mental tests and an autopsy of the mind after death. Researchers determined that small blood vessel disease accounted for approximately 1/three of the threat of dementia within the 221 autopsies finished. Importantly, for some time, this shape of ailment of small blood vessels may match neglected. They do now not speak approximately huge things like a stroke or blood clot that blocks a huge artery. Such minor problems, however, can upload up over the years, fundamental to cognitive impairment.

This research, of path, comes from the Pacific Northwest, the birthplace of grunge-rock and coffee from Starbucks. We can not make certain that these shape of humans don't have any post-angst cognitive sickness or reaction to a latent flannel blouse! Even after flooding the planet with highly-priced espresso, we cannot rule out laid low with a few shape of publish-annoying strain, equal to about $18.00 in keeping with gallon, marginally greater than we pay for gasoline. In reality, in Seattle, one humans (Evans) has been raised and may display some early symptomology.

Nonetheless, aside from the ones feasible confounds (The Powers is wrong and his faithful cronies invested carefully in Starbucks in the path of the length, this research is quite widespread pass demonstrating the variety of factors this could make a contribution to dementia. Much importantly, it encouraged that with the aid of the use of searching after way of lifestyles factors which could shield in the direction of vascular disease, you may appreciably lower your chances of developing dementia.

The benefit is that we have an amazing idea due to the reality blood vessels artwork to offer nutrients to active regions of the body! So in case your mind is active (which calls for strength) and you enhance your everyday vascular fitness via eating right and workout, the possibilities are that the risk of developing dementia from small vessel sickness can be drastically reduced. It need to now be said that paintings in this problem rely is ongoing, however common sense can also endorse that this is going to be proper.

Taken collectively, this illustrates a few giant motives why the location of workout and vitamins in mind health is so critical. To feed new brain circuits customary with the aid of learning and intellectual interest, it's far vital to attend to each the ones way of life elements to preserve a healthy blood supply and to create new blood vessels. When you forget about approximately approximately this element of mind health, you could almost restriction your functionality to benefit from neurogenesis and synaptogenesis because of many applications aimed inside the direction of preserving your thoughts more youthful.

Memory Improvement Leads to a Healthy Lifestyle

Strengthening our reminiscence isn't a undertaking, and studying beneficial suggestions for improving memory isn't always for anyone at all. Memorization can be hard most of the time, however it could be advanced, and beneficial memory capability may be preserved. I endorse that you check some recommendations for improving your reminiscence so that you can decorate your way of lifestyles and memory. In my view, nicely health and an high-quality reminiscence are one of the primary keys to a a fulfillment lifestyles. Understanding and expertise how our body and thoughts works may also need to make a real difference to our perspective of the manner we stay our lives.

As they may be saying, "Knowledge is Power," and in case you need to live a long term, studying a manner to live healthily is a want to!

There are loads of thoughts for boosting fitness and reminiscence that we're capable of think about, but you need to realize the critical pointers.

For instance, consuming end end result and vegetables each day or at least 5 to six days in step with week, ingesting healthful food is crucial for our health. Blueberries, Raspberries, avocados, tomatoes, and strawberries, are beneficial as you try to preserve your thoughts balanced. A wholesome brain in the way you live and experience will deliver stability to your lifestyles and top notch strength. Please bear in mind the ones tips for enhancing your memory and workout what you recognize to your lifestyles, recollect your fitness, and the way stunning existence is, now not to attend to it.

Of starters, your mind desires to eat end result which might be considerable in antioxidants, at the side of cranberries, as it will maintain it healthy. Tuna, shrimp, salmon, and some seafood also are very useful in enhancing memory. You are taking already a large step inside the direction of a healthy lifestyle with the aid of including stop end result and greens in your diet and contributing to precise health. Creating your weight loss plan isn't difficult. Try that!

The awesome suggestions for reinforcing reminiscence are those you locate fun to do. At all times, try to preserve a amazing thoughts-set and mind, and you can gather the farthest dreams.

Okay, now, whilst you're making your weight-reduction plan, make certain you have got were given fruit and vegetables every day or 4-five days in keeping with week, at least! Try slicing again on terrible meals and junk meals. This will not do any harm occasionally, however ultimately, you may apprehend how risky this type of meals may be on your body.

It's additionally essential to devour meat, so make sure you consume your burger as a minimum once each week. Or you can visit IHop with a salad at the facet and an entire cup of bloodless water, get your self the T-bone steak. If that could make it less complicated for you, it would art work as properly, however commonly selfmade meals is better and greater secure, of direction.

The first step to a exchange you are inclined to make on your life want to be to write down down down and create a healthful diet for your self. It's a massive soar forward!

So skip and get a pad, pen/pencil, and consider a weight loss plan that is going to go together with you, bear in mind stop result and greens on every occasion!

At all times, try to keep a incredible mind-set and thoughts. Seek it, as a minimum!

Now that you're extra snug along side your new diet, it's time to recollect doing bodily sports activities every day or as a minimum three to four days every week. Come on, lazy days; workout goes to carry power on your existence. Exercising moreover plays a vast function in our lives, alongside thing a proper diet. This improves our mind characteristic, allowing you to assume in reality approximately what is going to help you live pleasant continuously.

So, the following concept would be to attempt to make as a minimum four-five days every week a exercising agenda.

It's time to create a touch everyday of workout and add it on your every day time table. Training each day for as a minimum 10 to 15 minutes or at the least three to four days every week is a notable way to stay in form and keep a healthful mind with a wholesome frame. You need to do ten to twenty leaping jacks on Saturday, as an instance, to be able to in all likelihood take no greater than 3 to 4 minutes, after which you could stretch for five to 10 mins. Do this every morning, in real and healthful meals, it's going to start your day. You can change it a chunk and do exceptional sports activities.

Concentration and Its Effect on Memory Improvement

Concentration has an effect on memory recovery, due to the reality the name indicates. Improving your power is a way to decorate your reminiscence. Focusing right right here is the answer. You want to attention on what you are doing or wondering to pay attention absolutely. Concentrating permits in memorizing, and concentrating can also additionally have made you obtain this tons better at the equal time as you want to attempt to recall some specific type of facts.

The superb statistics I've were given for you is that hobby is a highbrow capability that you could develop yourself. Now the techniques you may enhance strength are twofold: First, regardless of the state of your environment, you need to try to growth the extent of awareness ability of your mind. In one of a type terms, try to pay more interest than traditional.

Firstly, create the high-quality environment for you to cognizance a bargain more quick. It is critical to create a appropriate environment in case you take part in an interest that requires entire attention. For example: looking for to memorize a poem.

Brain waking up: The awareness enhancement gadget can take a piece of try and energy, however it could no matter the reality that be some thing well certainly well worth doing. Some check a distinction in their functionality in best a short location of time to pay hobby.

Several books with reference to neuro-plasticity say that the way the character mind is ready and operating isn't always set in stone as scientists have continually believed. Quite the opportunity, every time you examine some thing new like a information, analyze by using coronary heart the similarly information, or improve the techniques you do things, the connections of your thoughts and neurons are hassle to alternate and improvement.

This locating is quite first rate in itself, because it gives in addition proof that your thoughts's capability to attention in a way this is already a fulfillment can despite the fact that be similarly extra suitable. However, those changes do now not take effect immediate, in accordance to research. You should hold strolling on it regularly for changes to begin showing up because of the reality what you are doing is reforming your mind.

Probably a question you've got got now could be how I can start to enhance my attention? What are the simplest techniques?

An approach to that is to attempt to in form your every day time desk with new conduct, that allows you to in addition increase the strength of your thoughts. Some of these behaviors are video video games that also beautify your hobby: the greater sure abilties are used, the greater their impact on the thoughts is indicated by means of way of research. So, concerning this, playing interest-based totally simply games and proper now video video video games will enhance your concentration's typical basic overall performance.

Adopting a wholesome way to choose the elements you devour: to pay hobby efficiently, the correct nutrients have to receive for your mind. It requires right blood sugar regulation as glucose is your thoughts's maximum critical nutrient.

Meditation: Try meditating instances a day, approximately five inside the morning, and every one-of-a-kind five within the nighttime in advance than going to sleep. If you're new to meditation, "The Miracle of Mindfulness: The Complete Guide to Meditation by way of manner of way of the Most Revered Master of the World."

Sleep and rest: It's critical to get loads of sleep and rest because of the fact at the equal time as now not having hundreds of every, you could not be able to attention at the activities of your subsequent day that allows you to probably lead to beneath-performance to your behalf.

Creating the ideal environment: Create an surroundings that permits you to pay interest better whilst challenge an interest that wishes your hobby, aside from incorporating the above-defined behaviors into your each day time table.

By worthwhile yourself, enhance your motivation. If the activity you are doing isn't always really a laugh, but a few thing you're doing as it wants to be completed, then builds a praise for yourself in case you need to make you more added on as you maintain collectively along with your challenge. For example, in case your preferred comedy begins offevolved in an hour, tell yourself you need to finish your assignment so that you can watch the sitcom in an hour.

Thinking about the inspiring revel in to be able to take location in an hour will help encourage you further and make you experience higher at the identical time as you whole the challenge.

Avoid distracting your self. Put to a prevent any loud sounds that could distract you and trade your function if it is not important. You may be interested by locating out that easy and instrumental song gambling will have a tremendous impact on your attention. Thinking about the inspiring revel in to be able to take vicinity in an hour will help inspire you further and make you experience higher even as you complete the venture.

Avoid distracting your self. Put to a stop any loud sounds that could distract you and alternate your role if it isn't vital. You may be interested by locating out that easy and instrumental tune gambling could have a excessive brilliant impact for your reputation.

The human mind is broadly identified to experience regular. Specialize an area to your environment to keep your hobby-related activities. Try to make it a dependancy of preserving the overall overall performance of the equal types of sports activities each time inside the same location. Stop acting duties like your hobbies in areas in which your thoughts and body are used to other subjects. For instance: for your dwelling room in which your family is gathering to look at television as this will purpose you to lose cognizance. The human mind is extensively recognized to revel in recurring. Specialize a place for your environment to store your awareness-associated sports. Try to make it a addiction of retaining the overall overall performance of the same varieties of events whenever inside the same vicinity. Stop appearing obligations like your hobbies in regions in which your mind and body are used to various things. For example: in your dwelling room in which your family is collecting to observe tv as this can purpose you to lose awareness.

The effect of colors on reminiscence: it is able to even sound unusual or bizarre, but colorations have an impact at the human thoughts in line with a file! Greenlight, for one, in keeping with a current have a check, increases popularity. So, buy the ones green bulbs and use them even because it's dark and if the inexperienced mild does not paintings, get crimson as an opportunity!

Chapter 11: Can You Reverse Memory Loss?

Overage, the majority of humans enjoy reminiscence loss. Yet psychologists discover that it's far often viable to correct those problems.

If human beings sense their reminiscences fading, they panic. The lawmaker, 68, have end up frenzied. He made embarrassing mistakes now, lengthy satisfied along with his functionality to take into account the names, the decision of the kids, and even the birthdays of giant substances. His reminiscence turned into now not what it was as soon as. Devastated, at a reminiscence hospital close to Seattle, he modified into looking for assist. Can the ones lapses in reminiscence be reversed? Was his future at danger? God forbid, is Alzheimer's sickness inside the early stages?

People panic once they experience their memories fading. Highly knowledgeable human beings have a propensity to panic once they suppose their minds are slipping in traumatic jobs. We have visible physicians, attorneys, company executives, and other lively human beings come to us for help. They're well aware about the ones shortcomings, and they're stressful." Recent research is helping to say those fears. While it is real that maximum humans begin to revel in a loss of their capability to don't forget subjects in their 50s and 60s, it's far now understood that this deterioration is seldom a sigh for neurological issues like Alzheimer's sickness. Memory loss, in maximum instances, outcomes from healthful mind modifications as well as cognitive adjustments that generally rise up with developing older. The right records is that there are techniques to rejuvenate memory for max people.

Medications decorate memory in people, extra than a dozen drug treatments were proven in U, which includes primates. S. Laboratories to enhance animal memory, collectively with primates. Human volunteer medical trials inside the period in-between are below ay, and findings are due in a few years. But for now, handiest one examined method is available to contrary memory loss: analyzing. Just as physical exercise counteracts the consequences of growing antique on the body, it enables to maintain the thoughts fairly intact. Studies have verified that if an character is stimulated sufficient, the ones techniques are quite useful.

Many Who Have Difficulty Recalling Conclude They Have Alzheimer's Most humans who've hassle remembering statistics bounce to the belief that they've Alzheimer's, a disorder that steadily saps memory, important to severe confusion and disorientation ultimately. Yet epidemiological research have verified that most effective 2 percentage of humans the various a while of sixty 5 and 75 are probable to boom the ailment. That technique ninety eight out of a hundred humans whose names, purchasing lists, and records are forgotten at the age of sixty five have everyday, balanced brains in magazine.

Neuroscientists now see learning and reminiscence as a dynamic approach that sculpts and re-sculpts within the mind, referred to as neurons, the connections among nerve cells. Some of those cells go through molecular adjustments every time a memory is laid down that both reinforces or weakens their contact with different neurons. If a person forgets some aspect, it most likely way that some of the hyperlinks are compromised or damaged.

These styles may be carried out to the three critical types of reminiscence: extended-time period, number one, and secondary. Long-time period reminiscence (diagnosed by using the usage of scientists as a ways flung reminiscence) includes records this might be to be saved for an entire life. Significant sports inclusive of a automobile crash or a little one's notion are mapped indelibly into the neural circuitry of 1.

Primary memory involves information-for example, a string of numbers which encompass a telephone range that is saved in our attention of attention nice in short. Our potential to copy a mobile phone variety is hardly ever declining with age right now after being attentive to it.

But secondary reminiscence is inclined-the capability to keep records beyond a few moments ' spans. Secondary reminiscence emerge as what "helps you to consider in that you parked the motor," that is growing drug-restoring reminiscence. "But you don't need to bear in mind every vicinity you have got got ever parked your automobile." That's why the mind is stored lengthy enough-minutes, hours, or days-to be beneficial after which forgotten.

According to David Arenberg, a psychologist on the National Institute of Aging, age impacts secondary memory extra than the Other Kinds humans of their 60s do no longer perform in addition to more younger human beings on just about every secondary memory check ever designed. For instance, on assessment, a listing of 12 phrases is proven to people, and after five mins, they'll be asked which phrase they could do not forget. Sixty-three hundred and sixty five days-olds aren't as excessive as 30-365 days-olds. Besides, people in the ongoing observe of the institute display a constant decline while re-attempting out every six years.

A panel of experts has named this phenomenon at countrywide health institutes: age-associated memory impairment. Some findings into its origins have arisen during the last decade from brilliant advances in neuro-sciences. Concerning neurochemistry, reminiscence loss associated with age, and the early tiers of Alzheimer's sickness is really indistinguishable. It may additionally moreover flip out that dementias together with Alzheimer's are exacerbated manifestations of natural ageing. Still, in some instances, it's miles doubtful how the cycle runs amok, and in others, it is particularly benign. Nor do scientists understand a way to age greater than exclusive kinds of memory have an effect on secondary reminiscence.

Most Neurons Shrink and Atrophy With Age: An Outdated Notion Researchers as quick as claimed that the death of an expected a hundred,000 neurons each day triggered memory loss. Yet stronger neuron counting techniques reversed the notion. It now appears that while some neurons die in regions of the thoughts which can be crucial for memory, the loss is more than a hundred cells in keeping with day. According to Larry R. Squire, a neuroscientist at San Diego Veterans Administration Medical Center, those deaths increase over 5 to six many years, and cellular loss can also additionally account for some of the memory deterioration that consists of getting older. But possibly a extra critical element is that with age, most neurons weaken or atrophy. It takes area because of a discount inside the improvement of materials called growth factors, which nourish neurons, in line with one hypothesis. Although those cells however perform, they've fewer connections to brilliant neurons.

Another concept elements to adjustments in chemistry. Chemicals referred to as neurotransmitters flow into backward and forward at the give up of the nerve among neurons, allowing the neurons to have interaction. Changes in the ones neurotransmitters ' diploma s can be in part answerable for the age-associated memory loss. Studies have backed this principle. Researchers have been able to reason the forms of memory lapses frequently suffered thru way of sixty five-yr-olds in 25-12 months-olds with the useful resource of giving capsules to more younger human beings that inhibit the interest of cholinergic compounds, a fixed of reminiscence-essential neurotransmitters. Their minds lower back to ordinary whilst the medicine wore off.

Many prescription drugs taken thru way of many older humans may additionally moreover have a comparable deleterious impact. The remedy right right right here is straight forward: to exchange the drug ordinary of the affected person.

Medications for Improving Memory For Available In Europe Scientists argue that if chemical modifications in the mind result in reminiscence loss, it may be counteracted with the beneficial aid of chemical substances within the shape of medicinal tablets. There are really more than 20 drug treatments available in Europe to beautify reminiscence, but they have got no longer been examined under the rigorous standards of America. So a long manner, within the United States, simplest one drug, Hydergine, has been approved.

There is the motive for optimism, however. Experiments have shown that medications can beautify the memories of strong vintage monkeys. Other experiments have tested that the same types of memory loss human experience as monkeys. It is reasonably-priced to trust that they'll additionally be reversible in humans if such issues may be reversed inside the monkey.

No Criteria When Thomas Crook created the Memory Assessment Clinics in 1985, one in every of his pastimes changed into to check different capsules that have been idea to have the capability to recover reminiscence. However, he emerge as confronted with a trouble: few wholesome people were ever tested for memory function, so there are not any requirements or baselines to distinguish some of the memory losses due to getting older. Such differentiation turn out to be critical in order that the medication is probably examined accurately. Crook conjectured that some medicinal tablets would possibly advantage people whose recollections are suffering from contamination, but now not humans with an first-rate memory, or vice versa. He first needed to increase baselines to decide which medicinal pills are suitable for which situations.

Computer administers Crook's New Memory Tests, But the reminiscence characteristic tests to be had have been old and beside the factor to normal existence problems. So, a few new necessities have been set up with the useful resource of manner of Crook and his colleagues. The checks are done through masses of volunteers, who measure the potential to remedy such regular reminiscence problems as figuring out missing gadgets and recalling names. These check outcomes have shed mild on the everyday and peculiar loss of reminiscence. For instance, consistent with Crook, humans with healthy reminiscence loss will be predisposed to misplace items, however they now not often wander away within the occasion that they retrace their steps alongside a acquainted street. Losing one's manner may be an Alzheimer's symptom in familiar territory. Once baselines were identified, a whole lot of memory-improving drugs had been evaluated via the clinics.

Blood strain drug treatments can beautify memory as a thing impact Some excessive blood stress prescription drugs commonly usually have a tendency to beautify memory as a side effect and are being tested in human beings with ordinary blood strain. Substances known as phospholipids also are being studied, which can be idea to assist neurons absorb chemical substances that are important to reminiscence. Cortex's Raymond Bartus notes that in the laboratory, numerous cholinergic compounds have confirmed promise. But the ones trials are nonetheless within the early tiers, so it's far likely to be years earlier than the authorities approves any new memory drugs. And both Crook and Bartus warn that a panacea is not going to be a drug. To correctly counter memory loss, it's also critical to cope with the emotional component of the problem.

The ordinary getting older technique creates a defeatist thoughts-set for plenty humans. They turn out to be convinced that their reminiscence is going down the tubes and that it is viable to make a have a study. A younger character who feels that he is lacking his vehicle keys, "I desire I had paid hobby," and he turns to his partner and asks, "Have you taken my keys?" It's now not a dramatic occurrence. The older person is much more likely to apprehend important loss as adverse. He or she says, "I'm dropping my mind." This may additionally end up a prophecy that fulfills itself. These also can bring about depression, which is believed to make a contribution to the dearth of memory.

Often older humans end up masses less worried physical further to mentally, ensuing in lots much less pushed end-to-surrender with the aid in their environment. This stimulation can be an crucial thing in maintaining the mind wholesome, consistent with Dr. Jermone Yesavage, a psychologist at Stanford University, and the dearth of it may have an effect on the biochemical techniques involved in reminiscence. In this context, reputation is type of a muscle: if it isn't exercised, it atrophies.

The first step is to growth self-self notion, but the technique to the ones troubles does now not start with reminiscence sporting sports that require a wonderful deal of motivation. A character ought to assemble self belief in himself first. She makes use of behavioral remedy to counteract awful stereotypes in trying to help humans with age-associated memory impairment. She attempts to make her patron understand that at the same time as they may be enhancements in memory in later lifestyles, you probably can regulate, and you can modify one's mind through striving difficult and paying hobby.

Consider Associating the Name of a Person with Something Concrete: Mental Imagery One set of memory-improving wearing occasions is based totally on highbrow imaging. The idea is to partner the selection of someone with a tangible component. You may be a part of the name to his superb nose with image of dollar bill. The photo will come to mind and be aware him the following time you notice him, the picture will start to min, and you'll do not forget his call. Dr. Yesavage examined the method on undergraduates from Stanford. "We will remember names like loopy inner 15 mins," he says.

Nevertheless, it's far greater tough for older people to accumulate a video library of pictures.

Once you have got developed landmarks, you're mentally setting a food object at every spot. You "stroll" along the road at the same time as it is time to maintain in thoughts groceries' listing and recollect that object as it is located. The interest is truely due to the fact you don't want to worry about the order of the matters and due to the fact the associations regularly provide compelling pics-bread loaf filled in mailbox or raisins spread along the corridor. Lists may be stored inside the reminiscence for about 24 hours the use of this shape.

How to apply unforgettable highbrow photographs of numbers Other pointers to keep in mind names are useful. You could probably use memorable highbrow pix for the numbers; might be twins, one is probably a pole, and 6 a % of beer. So, Flight 216 becomes a intellectual picture of twins putting from the pole consuming six packets or rhymes, and photographs may be utilized in conjunction: two and hat, one and moon, six and sticks. Flight 216 is a video of a shoe sitting close to a stack of stickers in the warm sun.

The mystery to successfully prosecuting reminiscence enhancement techniques is encouragement. Understanding that reminiscence loss is normally reversible is frequently sufficient to inspire human beings to do their remarkable.

The elderly Congressman had enough motivation: he knew his future changed into on the road, and remembering motivates a politician greater than dreaming of moving decrease lower returned to the location. The congressman can now don't forget names and faces in addition to he ever did with the beneficial resource of strategies acquired at the clinic of Thomas Crook.

Easiest Way To Improve Memory

"Memory is the protector of all topics"- Cicero The brilliant capability during life to preserve the mind active calls for conscious attempt. In truth, what we loosely check with as memory is lots of numerous techniques taking place in the mind. It is feasible to interrupt up the concept of reminiscence into quick-time period memory and prolonged-term reminiscence. These are basically one in all a kind structures, even though they have interaction. Only a part of quick-time period memory can be have become lengthy-time period storage. The mind synthesizes protein for brand spanking new dendrites and axon pathways after figuring out whether or not or not an hobby it's miles witnessing is satisfactorily crucial for survival at the same time as an occasion happens within the long term. The mind's frontal lobes, hippocampus, and cortex are all actively involved inside the processing, preservation, and retrieval of records.

To be able to accomplice a present day reality with an vintage one is the key to building a memory capability that lasts. It is possible to keep our recollections alive and functioning. Imagine being at a meeting, and you're the best character who can recite the mission announcement of the corporation, accept as true with what a boost it's far going to be. It is possible to use severa techniques to preserve the reminiscence alive. By becoming continuously fascinated, a distracted mind can be jolted into movement. It permits the self-reputation and gives an aspect wherein others have did no longer tread; you will be there and be in advance-talk about the gain it brings. The use of mnemonics or reminiscence aids is some other shape.

Remember the letters used to memorize notes at the ACEG (All cows devour grass) bass clef, that is beneficial at the identical time as there may be a huge amount of memory committing information. All it has to do is to reflect with a letter a selected reality. At the start, you have got were given many notes that can be delivered collectively for brief don't forget in significant wholes. Only remind yourself of the addresses, and you have were given the records to your beck and talk to.

Remember a time, and I advise thrilled while you felt thrilled. Picture the apparel you've got been wearing, the people spherical you, the music inside the historical beyond, the perfume inside the air............... You might be smiling proper now!

Across unique areas, the hippocampus carries lengthy-term recollections. Mixed emotions normally will be inclined to save scenes within the mind, whether or now not fantastic or bad. Consciously, the usage of feelings permits to commit facts to reminiscence. Imagine yourself as you have been content material cloth fabric lower back within the nation; preserve your highbrow pics as clean as you could. In that cushty kingdom, devote a few problem to reminiscence. Return to that united states of america in your thoughts on the time of remembrance, see, you tricked your mind into storing a truth. This is specifically accurate for people going for getting, do that to dedicate an prolonged listing to memory. Arrange the gadgets in a totally insane manner, the Secret proper right here is creativeness, e.G., Secret, dolphin, boat, sand Imagine carrying a first rate key; insert it right right into a whale's element (think about the whale as an aircraft!) You flip the important thing and open an excellent whale's detail.

A large deliver strategies from the component of the whale, colliding with you because it makes the ocean so deep that it takes the whale with it. You get the important element, the whale, the supply, and the sand-you cannot stand at the water, of direction! The trick proper right here is to apply insane establishments-the following time you have got to shop for groceries, to prepare your things like this, you want to keep masses in mind with out losing any. Concentration is an important problem of education. It is an functionality that can be determined out to stay focused on a particular difficulty and now not allow hobby to waver. Sit down pretty certainly and though your mind, take deep breaths with every depend as you don't forget from 30, exhale.

After the workout, observe an item (perhaps a stone): look at the scale, contours, markings, gaps, weight, and a texture-paying attention to any feature it has and so well realize the item that if it's far combined with others, you would be capable of pick it up without any troubles. Now consider choosing up the object on your mind and going via the complete system. Do this for about 5 minutes-the precept idea here is to maintain your mind quiet and hobby on a specific challenge at a time. Over time, you come back to understand that instructions determined out on this america of the usa of the us have a propensity to paste faster, longer, and higher. "Let the inclined say I am sturdy" Infect your subconscious thoughts with regular excellent affirmations. It options up everything you are pronouncing and magnifies it.

Make it a addiction of continuously declaring and telling your self that you have a remarkable memory that is strong and effective; it's far going an extended way to keeping one mentally balanced. The subconscious thoughts is going to artwork and is helping to reinforce the declare. It simply changes the individual's mindset and instills self warranty. Strict academic, notwithstanding the reality that! It's an super method to chart minds. This involves breaking the information with the number one elements linked to the huge heading to be memorized into small bits.

Curiosity Memory Improvement Mnemonics Strong Emotions Creative Associations Affirmation Mind Mapping Repetition This is a easy pattern of a thoughts map; it is able to be greater complete relying on the statistics to be memorized. Constant repetition of sports already found out, playing again pics stored in mind permits to consolidate in addition getting to know material. Most of what is found is rapid forgotten if the principle hyperlinks are not revised constantly. If that is completed frequently, it's miles set for life by using manner of the hippocampus inside the term memory. In stop, "Repetition is the mother of functionality," exercising-exercising-practice.

Thinking Fast Isn't That Simple!

Have you ever wondered how coffee drives your thoughts into movement-and wherein with out it we might be? When it's time to assume quick, there may be no doubt that we people mechanically look for "steroids." The impulse is to wake up the neuropeptides in the cerebral cortex- and get them to bop in a flurry of polka.

Picture a thousand million steroidal peptides (neurochemicals) jumping and skipping madly, doing cartwheels and strolling on the pinnacle speed, zooming inside and out of the frightened machine's laneways and highways, never pausing for air-until unluckily, fatigue sets in.

That's even as you take note of the z's... Dozing... High after the coffee. After an overdose of dopamine, the peptides snoring in the path of the synapses and the adrenals flapping violently inside the air.

Coffee is appropriate for a fast chortle-it does the trick in case you want to get immoderate for a fast burst without being illegal. Thinking in a immediately line turns into as sincere as being pulled lower lower back at the floor via manner of an excellent rope walker. There are no longer obscure mysticism meanderings, or tries at intensity-conclusions are open and closed case-easy, concise, and unchallengeable.

Correctly why human beings use espresso so profoundly, so compulsively, it nonetheless seems like an thrilling thriller. It's recognized to be addictive-but. There's a darker, sinister motive why we need espresso tragically? Could it's due to the fact we misplaced the ability to expect concisely (without espresso)? Scary concept that I modified into going to say.

Without the morning snap-afternoon and night (let's get real proper right here), in that are we going to be? Would the extremely good performance at their edgy but be our revolutionary agencies of authors, musicians, and visual artists?

Would the area be a one of a kind area without the kick-a-bean that resorts with out troubles in our cranium to hold the wheels of commercial enterprise spinning? The sweat of the strolling magnificence maintains pumping-and the relaxation people supply deeply insightful insights to entertain us?

Coffee is a psychoactive drug, of course. It might not be openly admitted, however the opium-the seed of the opulent poppy-has a similar addictive quality. How paradoxical that we overdose on caffeine to count on simply.

Of direction, paradoxes abound-as a long way as addiction is concerned-however that, high-priced readers, is every other story whole of sound and, of route, fury. Was the question raised-being the end quit result of lengthy years of grinding and ingestion of coffee endemic anger? Clinical studies have established that stress, tension, or maybe panic assaults upward push in doses of three hundred milligrams or more in some individuals. We can't string mind within the morning with out it. With it, no matter the fact that, we can boom violent behaviors that would lead to lengthy-term tension — not a lovable story.

Used with patented coffee, consisting of perception, or maybe sturdiness will benefit the brain as it turns on the vital frightened device. Yet even as the body can not do with out it, the go-over aspect comes. When is it precisely? Is it the number one detail inside the morning whilst we cry out to our lover-earlier than the ritual drink? Or even as we in the long run supply in to the hunger in advance than we fall asleep... Many human beings may also want to anticipate that is flawlessly natural. It is, of direction, but best if depleted adrenals are not able to offer even a vulnerable signal to save you in addition self-annihilation.

Coffee has leaped effectively and maliciously into our culture-vehemently bent at the capability of humanity to anticipate without it to self-destruct. It's this kind of curse, although? Or is it simplest a shoulder to lean on for a while we accumulate our thoughts hoping that any character will provide you with an opportunity as extremely good as possible.

And so, the dance maintains-every day, each day. Coffee machines spill the beans, and we drink in a hurry within the aroma. However, it only takes a second to be aware that the dance edges out of control, the students of the attention constrain, the races of the heart, the mind buzz anxiously, and we are speakme-oh how we're talking!

Talk is fairly-priced, of path. The extra we communicate, the extra we recognize that there may be no longer some thing however warm air to endure in mind itself. And that warmth air is flowing over cafes, eating places, and shops in which coffee machines keep spilling the beans, anxiously looking forward to increasingly more customers, keen to consume.

The coffee demon sends customers to the espresso shops in which they lean lower lower back happy-and relax for that brief 2nd. It's a 2nd of rest-preventing and mastering, or just searching the area skip with the aid of.

The amusing part of ingesting coffee is to prevent and watch. It feels expert, and doing the "proper" issue-it looks as if a sanctuary and an enjoy for the own family. It's a few thing we have to love in our tradition-sitting in small cafes and playing the agency of each awesome even though it is a bit distance away.

So, there is coffee with us! Doesn't that perform a bit issue?

Coffee is a bane and a blessing-wherein with out it at this point, may want to the industrialized worldwide be? Would we've got had the focus to discern out wherein machines are going to telepath with our mind short? Then they'll discover what shape of thoughts-and at the burnt bean, devoted to crema, devoted to the sound. Ultimately, will espresso rule the arena as we as fast as felt we have been ordering laptop structures? Can our excited thoughts specific that coffee is a wonderful hassle to start the morning with the brand new pc structures? And what then.